POPE PIUS XII LIB., ST. JOSEPH COLLEGE
3 2528 01335 2309

ADDICTION IN THE NURSING PROFESSION
Approaches to Intervention and Recovery

Mary R. Haack, R.N., Ph.D., C.A.C. is Associate Director for Research at Northwestern University Center for Nursing, Chicago, Illinois, and a Guest Researcher at the National Institutes of Health, Bethesda, Maryland. She received her B.S.N. in 1974 from Loyola University of Chicago and her M.S. in 1980 in Psychiatric Nursing and Ph.D. in Nursing Science in 1985 from the University of Illinois.

She has served as a board member of the Illinois Nurses Association, Peer Assistance Network for Nurses (PANN) and is a member of the National Nurses Society on Addictions (NNSA), the Drug and Alcohol Nursing Association, Inc. (DANA), the Research Society on Alcoholism, and the Kettil Bruun Society for Social and Epidemiological Research on Alcohol. She has chaired the Nursing Research and Practice Section of the International Council on Alcohol and Addictions (ICAA) since 1980. She is affiliated with the American Nurses Association and Sigma Theta Tau (Alpha Lambda Chapter).

She is currently the recipient of a Clinical Investigator Award from the National Center for Nursing Research to study panic disorder among adult children of alcoholics. The study is being conducted at the National Institute on Alcohol Abuse and Alcoholism, National Institutes of Health, Bethesda, Maryland.

Tonda L. Hughes, R.N., M.S.N. received her A.S.N. and B.S.N. degrees from Eastern Kentucky University in Richmond, Kentucky. She earned a M.S.N. in Psychiatric and Community Mental Health Nursing from the University of Kentucky, Lexington, Kentucky and is currently completing work for her Ph.D. (Nursing Sciences) degree at the University of Illinois at Chicago. Ms. Hughes is currently a research assistant for the Women's Health Concentration at the University of Illinois at Chicago and Assistant Editor for the journal *Women's Health Nursing Scan* published by J.B. Lippincott.

Ms. Hughes holds memberships in the American Nurses Association, Sigma Theta Tau, Midwest Nursing Research Society, National Nurses Society on Addictions, Association for Women in Psychology, International Council on Women's Health and the International Council on Alcohol and Addictions.

She is a board member of the Illinois Peer Assistance Network for Nurses (PANN), a member of the Illinois Organization of Nurse Executive's Task Force on the Impaired Nurse, and the Illinois Professional Assistance Programs Consortium. Her research interests include women's mental health, women and addiction, and chemical dependency in the nursing profession. Ms. Hughes' research on Chief Nurse Executives' Responses to Chemically Dependent Nurses is funded by Sigma Theta Tau (Alpha Lambda) and the Illinois Hospital Association.

Addiction in the Nursing Profession

Approaches to Intervention and Recovery

Mary R. Haack, R.N., PH.D., C.A.C.
Tonda L. Hughes, R.N., M.S.N.
Editors

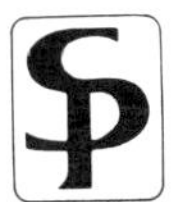

SPRINGER PUBLISHING COMPANY
NEW YORK

To my children,
Stephen, Jennifer, and Peter Haack
for their loyalty and affection.

To my parents, Ruby and Earl Hughes,
thanks for always believing in me
and for encouraging me to strive
for higher levels of accomplishment.

Springer Publishing Company, Inc.
536 Broadway
New York, NY 10012

89 90 91 92 93 / 5 4 3 2 1

Library of Congress Cataloging-in-Publication Data

Addiction in the nursing profession : approaches to intervention and recovery / edited by Mary R. Haack and Tonda L. Hughes.
p. cm.
Includes bibliographies and index.
ISBN 0-8261-6150-2
1. Nurses—Substance use. 2. Substance abuse—Treatment.
I. Haack, Mary R. II. Hughes, Tonda L.
[DNLM: 1. Nursing. 2. Substance Abuse—rehabilitation. WM 270 A2236]
RC564.5.N87A32 1989
362.2'9'088613—dc19
DNLM/DLC
for Library of Congress 88-24961
CIP

Printed in the United States of America

Contents

Foreword

The existence of chemical impairment in nursing is not surprising. What is surprising is that as a profession we claimed responsibility for the problem when it was not popular to do so. We are indebted to those nurses who came forward publicly, breaking the silence about their impairment and subsequent progress toward recovery. They gave us hope and a movement was born.

Because we were concerned about the chemically impaired nurse, my colleagues and I at the Nell Hodgson Woodruff School of Nursing at Emory University were moved to sponsor the First National Symposium on the Impaired Nurse in 1982. This symposium was the first open forum at a national level on the topic of impairment and served to establish the beginning of a network that has continued to work for the common good of society, the impaired nurse, and the nursing profession. The participants of these conferences, now held annually, are demonstrating that there is "help through hope" for nursing impairment related to chemical dependency.

Addiction in the Nursing Profession: Approaches to Intervention and Recovery provides another milestone. Now, for the first time, recognized nurse experts have been brought together to share their "state of the art" thinking, experience, and research findings in a collection of chapters on the subject of impaired nursing practice.

The book is organized in a logical sequence. The reader is informed of the scope of the problem and subsequently has an opportunity to read about several approaches to the development of programs to assist the chemically dependent nurse. It provides the reader with a comprehensive view of the issues arising from this problem. Such issues are related to the nurse, the profession, and the public. The publication of this work makes possible wider distribution of information important in the development of more effective and humane methods of assistance for our chemically impaired colleagues.

The editors and many of the contributors of this volume are recognized through their presentations, publications, and research as experts and pioneers in the study and care of the nurse whose professional functioning is impaired by chemical dependence.

I am honored to write the Foreword to this important publication and am confident that it will help readers in their research and practice.

Rose C. Dilday, M.A., R.N.
Professor Emeritus
School of Nursing
Nell Hodgson Woodruff
Emory University
Atlanta, Georgia

Introduction

Although use of the term "impairment" to describe incompetent or substandard practice caused by abuse of chemical substances is relatively new, impairment is not a new phenomenon. Like other social phenomena that remain elusive until publicly recognized and labeled, impairment among nurses was largely ignored until the late 1970s. Furthermore, although articles and position papers on the subject have recently begun to proliferate, data regarding impairment among nurses are still limited and inconclusive.

While there are a number of reasons for the dearth of information on chemical dependency in nurses, three appear to be particularly salient. First, it is difficult to conduct research on problems that are stigmatized by society and for which denial is a characteristic defense. Second, this difficulty may be compounded in nurses, who because of their professional socialization and fear of professional and legal reprisal may be more reluctant to disclose problems of personal substance abuse or to deal with such abuse by colleagues. Third, and perhaps most important, organized nursing has only recently begun to acknowledge chemical dependency as a significant problem and one for which the profession has some responsibility (ANA, 1982).

When impaired practice threatens the standards of health care delivery, action at the individual, institutional, and professional levels is necessary to protect the client, the nurse, the health care institution, and the profession.

Prevalence of Chemical Impairment in Nursing

Although little research has been conducted in the area, it is widely reported that health professionals, particularly nurses and physicians, experience chemically related impaired functioning at a rate disproportionately higher than the general public (Caroselli-Karinja & Zboray, 1986; Fowler, 1986; Green, 1984; Smith & Seymour, 1985; Talbott, 1983; Winick, 1974, 1980). The American Nurses' Association estimates that about six to eight percent (about 120,000 to 160,000) of the registered nurse population has a drug- or alcohol-related problem (ANA, 1987).

The most concrete data concerning impairment in nursing come from actions taken by state licensing boards. In a 1981 survey of state boards of nursing, 35 of the 37 boards that responded regarded substance abuse as increasingly serious. A more recent survey of state licensing boards found that 67% of all disciplinary actions in 1985 were related to alcohol or drugs (Chesney, 1985, reported in Sullivan, Bissell, & Williams, 1988, p. 172). However, disciplinary hearings can be conducted only when nurses have been reported, and it is well documented that addicted nurses frequently are ignored, fired, or asked to resign rather than reported to state licensing boards (Bissell & Haberman, 1984; Isler, 1978; Jaffe, 1982; Jefferson & Ensor, 1982). Therefore, these data may reflect only a portion of the problem.

Whether the prevalence of impaired functioning caused by abuse of or addiction to chemical substances is more limited, or greater than what is reported in the literature, there is increasing recognition that the problem must be addressed. It is becoming more widely recognized that to ignore addiction among nurses not only denies the individual nurse much needed help and enables progression of the addictive process, but also places at risk patients and staff for whom the impaired nurse is responsible.

Coming to Terms with the Problem

The problem of drug abuse and addiction in the United States has been recognized and sporadically addressed throughout this century (e.g., the Harrison Act of 1914 and the Marijuana Tax Act of 1937); however, drug abuse was not a source of widespread public concern until the 1960s and early 1970s. This concern was reflected by the massive increase in the number of articles devoted to the subject between 1964 and 1971; in federal expenditures for treatment, research, and prevention, which rose tenfold; and in expenditures for law enforcement, which rose sevenfold during that period (Litz & Walker, 1980).

While the "drug scare" of the 1960s and the early 1970s began to dissipate by the middle to late 1970s, the problem of drug use and abuse in American industry and the professions has gained increasing attention during the 1980s. The current incidence and patterns of drug use and abuse have instigated a set of concerns different from those of earlier decades. In previous years many individuals viewed the problem as being limited primarily to "fringe" groups such as "hippies," musicians, ghetto dwellers, and racial minorities. The American public has been more reluctant to admit that those people who transport us, protect us, and care for us are also likely to use or be addicted to mind-altering substances.

Nevertheless, recent reports in our media reflect a problem in the business and health care fields of much greater magnitude than was previously recognized. Drug use and abuse in business and industry have reached such proportions that most major corporations offer benefits that include provision for drug and alcohol treatment, and many have developed employee assistance programs. For businesses, the recognition that employee health and performance have a direct impact on production is incentive enough to encourage open discussion and confrontation of the problem.

Within the health care profession, recognition of and response to the problem has come more slowly. For health professionals such as nurses and physicians, the very considerations that make it imperative to confront such problems and take prompt action make it more difficult to admit that the problem exists. That is, health professionals are often responsible for making decisions crucial to the lives and well being of others. Consonant with the seriousness of this responsibility, however, are health professionals' perceptions of themselves as invulnerable to addiction. Because their education and training instills in them the expectation that they provide care to others, that they be physically, mentally, and emotionally strong under conditions of severe stress, and that they understand the physiological consequences of drug and alcohol abuse, health care professionals believe that they can control their drug use. Ironically, because they often will not allow themselves to express emotions or admit mental and physical exhaustion, they may turn to readily available drugs or alcohol as a means of alleviating stress.

The general public has also been unwilling to accept that those who care for others have human limitations and might also need help themselves. Much of the reluctance to admit the vulnerability of health care professionals stems from negative stereotypes and a lack of accurate information concerning alcoholism and drug addiction that have existed in the United States for decades.

While there has been some shift in attitudes toward a more rehabilitative approach to treatment in the past decade, the current financial upheaval in the American health care system has already begun to influence the allocation of monies for treatment of addictions. In a time of spiraling health care costs, it is not surprising that there is an increasing emphasis on responsibility for one's own health and a decreasing willingness to expend resources on problems believed to be caused by a lack of individual will. In addition, the burgeoning growth of malpractice cases over the past decade has caused increasing concern among hospital administrators about liability for the risks involved in employing nurses and physicians whose professional functioning is chemically impaired.

These factors, as well as an overall heightened interest in, and scrutiny of, professional standards (Kaplin, 1976) influence significantly the reaction to impairment of nurses and other health professionals in the United States.

Professional Responses to Impairment

Over the past decade, most health care professions have established programs to assist members whose practices are impaired by alcohol, drugs, or by psychiatric illness. The philosophical basis for these programs is humanistic concern, which a mature profession demonstrates for the well-being of its members, as well as the responsibility a profession has to society to self-regulate the practices of its membership to assure quality professional practice (ANA, 1984).

Programs for the impaired physician have been in place since 1976. The American Medical Association (AMA) presently operates its own Department of Substance Abuse out of its headquarters in Chicago. This department publishes the AMA Impaired Physician Newsletter, sponsors an annual conference on impairment among health professionals, disseminates information about support groups, state medical society programs and services, produces audiovisual materials, and publishes a directory of treatment facilities. In addition, the AMA provides information to concerned spouses and significant others.

Programs for nurses were initiated following a resolution passed by the American Nurses' Association (ANA) at its convention in 1982. This resolution called for (1) the development of guidelines for use by state nurses' associations and in creating programs of care for the impaired nurse, (2) the education of nurses, administrators, and employers regarding issues and rights of nurses who are impaired, and (3) the ongoing collection and dissemination of information on prevalence, programs, education, research, and ethical issues related to the impaired nurse.

The progress made since 1982 is significant, but each advance brings a deeper awareness of the complexity of the issue. Although psychological dysfunction is included in the ANA resolution, relatively little effort has been made to meet the needs of the nurse impaired by conditions other than substance abuse and dependence. The medical profession is just beginning to explore the issue of suicide prevention and strategies for dealing with psychiatric impairment among physicians.

When a nurse develops a substance-dependence problem there are numerous professional, social, and physical consequences. The most powerful influence in minimizing these consequences is the active involvement of colleagues, administrators, and professional organizations. The caring and skillful intervention of the professional community is necessary to assure nurses that they are deserving of treatment.

Addicted nurses seldom volunteer for treatment. The nurse who is confronted with documented dysfunctional behavior may be angry, defensive, or ashamed. These feelings make everyone involved uncomfortable. Confrontation is usually necessary and must often involve family, co-workers, and supervisors. Without the powerful statement made by such a confrontation, many nurses now in recovery would have persisted in denying their problem. This experience leaves them feeling exposed and vulnerable. How could they have failed their patients? How could they have failed their colleagues? How could they have failed their profession? And lastly, how could they have failed themselves? Those in administrative positions who provide support and direction in this time of crisis are essential to the successful entry into treatment and ultimate recovery of the nurse. The nursing administrator is key in establishing the expectation that treatment and demonstrated recovery are stipulations of continued employment. This issue is covered in Chapters 7 and 10.

Attitudes of nursing administrators and colleagues are critical to the successful implementation of any policy designed to help the impaired nurse. These issues will be discussed in Chapters 1, 2, and 12. The nurse who is impaired is usually in no position to choose a rehabilitative program, so those who confront the nurse must also design the program of treatment, or at least have a treatment evaluation scheduled. The nurse can then be given the responsibility of agreeing to it or refusing it. Chapters 3, 4, 5, 6, and 11 address the issues related to treatment options.

Assuming the role of patient or client is particularly difficult for the nurse, whose identity as caregiver is integral. Treatment programs designed to rehabilitate health professionals recount how nurses in treatment neglect their own needs in order to respond to fellow patients. The nurse–patient relationship that is so much a part of nursing socialization is, after all, a nonreciprocal one. For this reason the treatment of the nurse requires special considerations.

The recovery process is sometimes lengthy and arduous for health professionals who have subjugated their own needs to those of others for such a long time and in such dysfunctional ways. Part of the recovery plan may require that the nurse delay returning to the clinical setting for some time so that a firm, well-grounded recovery can begin.

In the recovery process, the nurse also frequently confronts a career crisis. Why was nursing chosen as a profession in the first place? Will continued practice of nursing facilitate or jeopardize the prospects for recovery? If the nurse is to remain in the profession, what new insights must be developed in order to function healthily as a nurse? Ideally, the programs that treat nurses offer opportunities to discuss these questions in groups where mutual support and problem solving can occur. Support groups and self-help groups for the recovering nurse are discussed in Chapters 8 and 9.

While there have been many program developments in the past decade that address the problem of impairment, the successful implementation of any program depends on adequate financial resources. Likewise, the successful recovery of any substance-dependent person requires a continuum of care that meets the particular needs of that person. This treatment requires insurance and other benefits that are often lost to the nurse when a substance abuse problem is identified. Furthermore, some programs developed in the 1970s and early 1980s have lost their original funding and have either become defunct or changed significantly. The survival of the ongoing work described in this book is an important issue that must continue to be addressed by the profession.

We hope that this book will serve as a guide to our colleagues in nursing in reaching out to impaired nurses. They are too valuable to the profession to lose.

TONDA L. HUGHES, R.N., M.S.N.
MARY R. HAACK, R.N. Ph.D.

Acknowledgements

Special recognition goes to Marilyn Fox, Ph.D., who served as technical editor for the first several drafts of this book. In addition, we are grateful to the faculty of the Women's Health Concentration at the University of Illinois at Chicago and to the Division of Biometry and Epidemiology, National Institute on Alcohol Abuse and Alcoholism for their enthusiasm and support throughout the development of this book.

References

American Nurses' Association. (1984). *Addictions and psychological dysfunctions in nursing: The profession's response to the problem.* Kansas City: Author.

American Nurses' Association. (1987, March). Impaired nursing practice (media backgrounder). *ANA News,* Kansas City: Author.

American Nurses' Association House of Delegates. (1982). *Action on alcohol and drug misuse and psychological dysfunctions among nurses.* Resolution #5, adopted June 29, 1982.

Bissell, L., & Haberman, P.W. (1984). *Alcoholism in the professions.* New York: Oxford University Press.

Caroselli-Karinja, M.F., & Zboray, S.D. (1986). The impaired nurse. *Journal of Psychosocial Nursing, 24*(6), 14–19.

Fowler, M.D. (1986). Doctoring or nursing under the influence. *Heart and Lung, 15*(2), 205–207.

Green, P.L. (1984). The impaired nurse: Chemical dependency. *Journal of Emergency Nursing, 10*(1), 23–26.

Isler, C. (1978). The alcoholic nurse: What we try to deny. *RN, 41*(7), 48–55.

Jaffe, S. (1982). Help for the helper: First hand views of recovery. *American Journal of Nursing, 82*(5), 578–579.

Jefferson, L.V., & Ensor, B.E. (1982). Help for the helper: Confronting a chemically-impaired colleague. *American Journal of Nursing, 82,* 574–577.

Kaplin, W.A. (1976). Professional power and judicial review: The health profession. *George Washington Law Review, 44*(August), 710–753.

Litz, C.W., & Walker, A.L. (1980). *Heroin, deviance and morality.* Beverly Hills, CA: Sage.

Smith, D.E., & Seymour, R. (1985). A clinical approach to the impaired health professional. *The International Journal of the Addictions, 20*(5), 713–732.

Sullivan, E., Bissell, L., & Williams, E. (1988) *Chemical dependency in nursing. The deadly diversion.* Menlo Park, CA: Addison-Wesley.

Talbott, D. (1983, April). *The disabled doctor.* Presentation at the First National Symposium on the Impaired Nurse, Atlanta.

Winick, C. (1974). Drug dependence among nurses. In *Sociological factors in drug dependence.* Cleveland: CRC Press.

Winick, C. (1980). A theory of drug dependence based on role, access to and attitude toward drugs. In D. Lettieri (Ed.), *Theories on drug abuse* (pp. 225–235). Research Monograph Series, No. 30. Rockville, MD: National Institute of Drug Abuse.

Contributors

Carol Bowers, R.N., CCDN
Director, Impaired Nurse Program, Talbot Recovery System
Atlanta, GA

Anne M. Cantazarite, R.N., B.S.N.
Director, Intervention Project for Nurses and
Consultant, Dept. of Professional Regulation
Jacksonville, FL

Olga M. Church, R.N., Ph.D.
Professor, The University of Connecticut School of Nursing
Storrs, CT

Suzanne Durburg, R.N., CNAA, M.Ed.
Associate Chair, Dept. of Nursing
Evanston Hospital
Evanston, IL

Pamela Billings Farley, R.N., M.S.N.
Assistant Professor, Dept. of Nursing
Berea College
Berea, KY

Janet Gaskin, R.N., M.S.N.
Director of Research and Program Development
The Donwood Institute
Toronto, Ontario, Canada

Patricia L. Green, R.N., M.S.W.
Chairperson, Impaired Nurse Committee
National Nurses' Society on Addictions
Evanston, IL

Lorraine Hall, R.N., M.N., M. Ed.
Manager of Health Services
Rhode Island Employee Assistance Program, Inc.
Warwick, RI

Marty Jessup, R.N., M.S.
Co-Founder, The Bay Area Task Force
Berkeley, CA

Beverly J. McElmurry, R.N., Ed.D.
Professor, College of Nursing
University of Illinois at Chicago
Chicago, IL

Madeline A. Naegle, R.N., Ph.D.
Associate Professor, Division of Nursing
Shimkin Hall
New York University
New York, NY

Jean Penny, R.N., Ph.D.
Continuing Education Director
Florida Board of Nursing
Jacksonville, FL

Judie K. Ritter, R.N., M.S.N.
Executive Director
Florida Board of Nursing
Jacksonville, FL

Ann Solari-Twadell, R.N., M.S.N.
President
National Nurses' Society on Addictions
Evanston, IL

Ruth R. Staten, R.N., M.S.N.
Assistant Professor
College of Nursing
University of Kentucky
Lexington, KY

Eleanor J. Sullivan, R.N., Ph.D.
Dean
School of Nursing
University of Kansas
Kansas City, KS

Jean Sullivan, R.N., B.A.
Co-Founder, Discovery
Seattle, WA

June Werner, R.N., M.S.N.
Chair, Dept. of Nursing
Evanston Hospital
Evanston, IL

Eileen Zungolo, R.N., Ph.D.
Associate Professor
College of Nursing
University of Illinois
Chicago, IL

1

Professional Issues, Ethical Constraints, and Legal Considerations

Madeline A. Naegle

Professional acts performed while the health professional is impaired have potential impact on society and the professional community. Traditionally, health professionals have been more highly valued and subject to closer public scrutiny than citizens employed in positions accorded lesser degrees of public trust. Society expects high levels of performance by health professionals because of their advanced education, clinical expertise, and access to personal aspects of citizens' lives. At the same time, unrealistic beliefs exist about the invulnerability of these professionals to certain diseases and behavioral states. Such notions are particularly evident in relation to drugs and alcohol, psychiatric illness, and cognitive impairment as a function of aging. When a health practitioner develops such an illness, the responses of the community span the continuum from denial to inhumane condemnation.

The balance between the rights of professional societies and organizations to regulate the practice of health professionals and the obligation to preserve public safety is not easily achieved. Since the 1960s, issues of professional responsibility, including licensure and state mandated legal regulation, have received greater attention. Three different but interrelated social perspectives can be used to view the problems of impaired practice: professional, ethical, and legal. Their interrelationship is implicit in the contract between society and a profession. Such a contract defines a mutually beneficial relationship that includes the delegation of authority to a profession to oversee vital functions and govern its own affairs. Self-regulation by the profession to assure quality performance is central to this contract. Professional organizations seek to fulfill their obligations through formulation and maintenance of professional standards, ethical codes, and the development of norms that sanction positive professional behaviors and identify negative behaviors as deviant.

Legal regulation of practice by health professionals derives from the delegation of responsibility for the public welfare to state governments. State boards of governmentally appointed individuals oversee the granting and revocation of licenses. Most frequently, these boards are composed of individuals who are members of the same professional discipline. The responsibilities and activities of professional societies, ethical constraints, and legal considerations must be clearly delineated in order to understand impaired nursing practice and its implications for professional communities and the public.

Impaired Nursing Practice as a Professional Issue

In the last thirty years, nursing has steadily progressed toward professionalism by planned internal change, newly defined relationships with other disciplines and clearer articulation of the relationship between societal needs and professional qualifications. The American Nurses' Association (ANA), recognized as the primary professional society, has relied on the expertise of its members to articulate a code of ethics and establish standards of practice. In addition, the organization promotes the development of nursing theory, establishes educational requirements for entry into the profession, develops certification processes, and implements projects related to nursing's professional accountability to the society (ANA, 1980).

In fulfilling its societal contract, nursing is granted the privilege of internal self-regulation. This means that the profession has a right to define and regulate standards of practice, to set educational requirements, and to articulate professional positions. The pursuit of the common good is related to provisions for the advancement of the profession's membership. Self-regulation of incompetent practice resulting from addiction, psychiatric illness, or cognitive deficits related to aging is subsumed within the provisions of the social contract. The preservation of public safety and welfare is central to the role of a profession; efforts to promote consumer well-being relate to that goal.

When a nurse practices at levels below minimal competence for a licensed professional nurse, standards of professional practice are seriously threatened. The nursing image projected is one of dangerous incompetence. Deficits in personal job performance, as well as failure to assume shared responsibilities, have impact on others in their attempts to deliver high quality nursing care. Standards of care are directly affected by the individual's unsafe practice or absence, and overall quality is compromised because others must compensate. This lowering of standards results in inconsistent or poor interpersonal care and may place the consumer at risk. Protection of the consumer and maintenance of standards are motivating forces for action at district, state, and national levels of nursing organizations.

In addition to self-regulation, the professional organization is committed to the economic and general welfare, including the professional well being, of its members. Organizational activity that promotes intellectual growth, professional advancement, health benefits, and work environments of limited risk to physical and mental health manifests such commitment. Changes within the health care industry are often spearheaded and supported by such activities, the overriding goals of which are improved working conditions and greater attention to health care needs. In states where the nurses' associations maintain units that act as bargaining agents for nurses in selected employment settings, such change is often produced through contract negotiations that address employment conditions. Of particular concern is the establishment of employment contracts that guarantee nurses health benefits and wages comparable to those of other professional employees. Benefits such as medical leave of absence and eligibility for disability payments are particularly important in relation to impaired practice. Treatment resources for substance abuse illness are frequently inadequate in program design and rehabilitation provisions for women. Few hospitals and health care agencies have employee assistance programs. When programs and health services do exist, nurses often do not use them. The reasons for this are unclear, but may relate to the absence of nursing staff in such settings, the too great visibility of the health service location, and a treatment approach that is less than professional and insensitive to the needs of a female population. Substance abuse counseling is often not available. Of further concern are the limitations of insurance coverage for hospitalization and rehabilitation services, including outpatient psychotherapy and addiction treatment.

Recognition of and response to problems of impaired nursing practice by professional organizations began in the late 1970s. Many of the initial efforts were by recovering nurses painfully aware of the stigma associated with being an addicted health practitioner and the lack of professional resources for support and direction into treatment. These efforts were supported by nursing specialty organizations such as the Drug and Alcohol Nurses' Association (DANA) and the National Nurses' Society for Addictions (NNSA), as well as by selected state nurses' associations. In 1978 the Maryland Committee for the Rehabilitation of the Nurse implemented the first "peer assistance program" in nursing. Modeled after similar programs established by medical societies, it consisted of outreach efforts and networks designed to motivate the health practitioner with impairment problems to discontinue practice and seek treatment and rehabilitation. Similar models were developed shortly thereafter in Tennessee, Ohio, and Illinois.

Program development became widespread when efforts to involve the American Nurses' Association at the national level were successful. In 1981 the Task Force on Addictions and Psychological Dysfunctions was convened. This group was composed of representatives of the ANA, the DANA, and the NNSA. The work of this group resulted in the formulation of a resolution adopted by the 1982 ANA House of Delegates: Resolution on Alcohol and Drug Misuse and Psychological Dysfunction Among Nurses. In subsequent years, the majority of state nurses' associations passed similar resolutions that support professional awareness and action on the problem. The task force also authored and edited a monograph on program development and salient issues related to the prevalence and nature of addictions and other dysfunctions that result in impaired practice.

The national resolution committed the ANA to establish mechanisms for disseminating information on the problem of impaired nursing practice, programs that address it, on educational and research efforts, and on legal and ethical issues. Further, it cited goals to educate employers and nurses and to provide guidelines for state program development. In stating these intentions, the action of the organization paralleled that of state medical societies, as well as groups in dentistry and pharmacy, that had identified the problem and had taken steps to organize formally. Beyond this, the national association assumed responsibility for providing leadership to state associations and other special interest groups within nursing and designated impaired practice an issue with broad ramifications for the profession, as opposed to a phenomenon affecting a few practitioners and of limited implications for others.

By 1978, 48 state associations had developed some type of program to assist nurses with alcohol or psychiatric problems or had designated committees to explore action plans (see Table 1.1). The types of programs currently operational include the following:

1. Information and Referral Services. Nurses, family members, coworkers or employers can obtain information on treatment or legal resources, can learn about disciplinary procedures, or be referred to crisis units and private practitioners. Some state nurses' associations maintain hotlines.

2. Formal Peer Assistance Programs. Groups of recovering and nonrecovering nurses, based with state nurses' associations respond to reports of an impaired colleague by outreach efforts that involve one-to-one contact, work with the family, or consultation to coworkers and employers. The goal of intervention is to motivate the individual into treatment. Noncoercive methods are the primary operating mode, but if the consumer is clearly endangered and the nurse refuses to respond to outreach efforts, state boards of nursing are contacted.

3. Peer Support Groups. Peer support activities take a variety of forms. State nurses' associations and specialty nursing organizations maintain a network of recovering individuals and other nurses in-

TABLE 1.1 State Nurses' Contacts Associations—

	Services offered						
	Intervention	Referral	Education	Peer Support Group	Contacts State-Wide	Re-entry Monitoring	Hotline
Alabama							
Alaska			•				
Arizona			•				
Arkansas							
California		•	•	•	•		
Colorado	•	•	•		•	•	•
Connecticut			•				
Delaware	•	•					
Dist. of Col.			•				
Florida		•	•				
Georgia	•	•	•	•	•	•	•
Guam							
Hawaii		•	•				
Idaho	•	•	•				
Illinois		•	•	•	•		
Indiana		•	•		•	•	•
Iowa							
Kansas	•	•	•		•	•	
Kentucky		•	•	•			
Louisiana	•	•	•		•	•	•
Maine							
Maryland		•	•		•		
Massachusetts		•		•	•		
Michigan		•					
Minnesota	•	•	•		•	•	
Mississippi		•	•				
Missouri		•	•	•	•		
Montana		•	•	•		•	
Nebraska	•	•	•	•		•	
Nevada			•	•			
New Hampshire	•	•	•				
New Jersey		•	•	•			
New Mexico	•	•	•	•			
New York			•		•		
N. Carolina		•	•		•		
N. Dakota		•	•				
Ohio	•	•	•	•	•	•	
Oklahoma	•	•	•	•	•	•	•
Oregon	•	•	•		•		•
Pennsylvania	•	•	•	•	•	•	
Rhode Island	•	•	•	•	•	•	•
S. Carolina	•	•	•	•	•	•	
S. Dakota			•			•	
Tennessee	•	•	•		•	•	•
Texas	•	•	•	•		•	•
Utah		•					
Vermont			•				
Virgin Islands							
Virginia		•	•	•	•		
Washington			•				
W. Virginia*	•	•	•	•	•	•	
Wisconsin							
Wyoming							

*Program independent of SNA

Peer Assistance Activities Overview

Assistance limited to		Program run by			Diversion legislation			
RN's only	Nurses who are state residents	Volunteers	Volunteers: expenses reimbursed	Paid staff	Passed		Considered	Rejected
		•		•			•	
•			•	•	•			
	•		•	•			•	
		•					•	
		•						
	•	•		•		•		
					•			
		•						
							•	
	•	•		•				
•	•	•	•	•				
			•				•	
•		•						
•		•	•				•	
•		•		•	•			
	•	•			•			
•			•	•			•	
•		•						
	•	•				•	•	
		•		•				
			•	•	•			
•	•	•		•			•	
		•						
			•	•				
	•	•	•	•				
		•					•	
			•	•				
	•							
	•	•						
	•		•					
	•		•	•	•			
	•	•					•	
		•					•	
	•	•						

terested in working with peers experiencing problems. Peer support groups that meet weekly in a variety of cities and regions assist nurses on issues central to recovery and the return to or maintenance of practice.

4. Education and Consultation Services. Individuals and groups in organizational and independent structures plan and implement educational programs in community and institutional settings. These programs are aimed at increasing levels of awareness of impaired practice, providing information on how to identify and intervene with a nurse who may have a drug, alcohol, or psychiatric problem and teaching strategies for the management of the problem in the employment setting. These offerings also emphasize the phases of reentry and the roles of nursing administrators, the recovering nurse, and nursing colleagues in implementing steps necessary for return to work.

In addition to the above models, collaborative models combine the resources of state nurses' associations and freestanding agencies. In at least two states, nurses' associations have established contracts for the provision of services by employee assistance programs. Volunteers on an association committee reach out to nurses and facilitate their entry into a treatment system by directing them to employee assistance programs where assessment and appropriate treatment recommendations take place.

Models in which collaboration among disciplines and with state boards for nursing also exist. In some states, nursing groups combine resources with medicine, dentistry, and pharmacy to create peer assistance for a multidisciplinary group. Not only does this approach contain costs and allow for more efficient use of knowledgeable personnel, but it fosters learning about problems that occur across disciplines and must be addressed by all health professionals.

Liaison relationships with state boards are recommended as a first step in program development. While the priorities of state boards for nursing and professional associations differ, the roles of both are essential to maintaining standards of nursing practice. State boards of nursing are responsible for disciplining practitioners for professional misconduct, and their actions result in censure and reprimand of the nurse, probationary status, or licensure revocation. Peer assistance can facilitate early intervention with an addicted or psychiatrically ill nurse, so that action by the state boards may not be necessary. Not infrequently, peer assistance moves the nurse to treatment before disciplinary action commences. In addition to the need for secondary interventions of identification and treatment, the profession recognizes the need for prevention. Education on health maintenance, stress management, and alcohol and drug use will ultimately change attitudes and support sanctions against alcohol abuse and other drug-using behaviors. Such education includes education on at-risk populations, the importance of cautionary use of alcohol to relieve tension or cope with distress and fatigue, adequate leisure activity, and the relationship of mental health to professional function. Students and practicing professionals need to understand the importance of monitoring the impact of drug use on practice, and the appropriateness of intervention when others are endangered. The profession's development of informal negative sanctions against impaired practice and education on its effect on professional role performance will ultimately provide deterrents. Change within the profession will produce resources for the prevention as well as the containment of the problem, thereby reducing the need for legal regulatory efforts.

Ethical Constraints

The professional education of nurses includes course content on ethics and ethical decision making. The ANA Code for Nurses provides ethical standards for the practice of nursing. While the code is clearly stated, in complex situations its implications are less straightforward and its interpretation strongly influences the choices for action on impaired practice.

When a colleague seeks to assist another nurse whose behavior suggests a dependence on alcohol and/or other drugs, ethical dilemmas often emerge. More than one ethical principle appears relevant, and appropriate courses of action may appear to conflict with one another. While the principle of beneficence may be clearly applicable in preventing harm to a patient, certain interventions may unfairly constrain a practitioner's right to autonomy. The goal may be the well being of a colleague, but interveners cannot always be sure that intervention does not violate the ethical principle of justice by wrongfully damaging another nurse's professional reputation.

One issue that often inhibits action is the lack of agreement on what constitutes "impaired practice." It has been stated that "nursing practice is impaired when the individual is unable to meet the requirements of the professional code of ethics and the standards of practice because cognitive, interpersonal or psychomotor skills are affected" (ANA, 1984). These phenomena may not be clearly evident, however, until the middle and late stages of addictive illness. Early intervention when impairment is less obvious is desirable for the practitioner's health and prognosis for recovery and is essential to prevent disciplinary action. Strategies used and the timing of intervention are affected, therefore, by individual circumstances as well as by ethical considerations.

Morrow (1984) discusses the importance of "blending of assistance and duress" in choosing strategies for intervention. The need for coercion should be based on considerations of at least three factors:

1. The substance abused and the victim of harm. Are individuals endangered or is harm to professional standards at issue?
2. Likelihood and immediacy of harm.
3. Severity of harm.

Such guidelines to identify the dimensions of harm assist the individual or group seeking a course of action to identify appropriate strategies. In situations in which the need for early intervention is indicated, personal suggestions or offers of assistance may be most feasible and effective. These are directed toward motivating the individual to seek treatment. While denial and other psychological barriers limit the potential for self-referral, such efforts may be the only ethically justifiable ones when the individual's ability to practice is in no way visibly affected. Social relationships and family life may be affected by heavy alcohol consumption, for example, but formal action cannot be justified until impairment is evidenced in job performance.

The ANA Ethical Code for Nurses, on the other hand, links formal action to impaired practice evidenced in behavioral change and poor job performance. The code designates peer responsibility for the health of another nurse and states that the nurse will "act to safeguard the client and the public when health care is affected by incompetent, unethical or illegal practice" (ANA, 1976). Conflicted personal feelings and an awareness of the consequences of licensure action, however, often influence ethical decision making and immobilize the practitioner so that no action is taken. Colleagues fear personal reprisal, legal action, and alienation from friends or coworkers if they express concern or report incidents or untoward circumstances to supervisory personnel. They often fear that action will violate the autonomy of a peer and unjustifiably label the person. Consultation in this type of decision making is invaluable and can enable the nurse to clarify circumstances, evaluate potential outcomes, and choose a course of action that both satisfies ethical constraints and provides assistance to the addicted or emotionally ill practitioner. Such consultation is available from individuals knowledgeable about impaired practice, representatives of peer assistance programs, district nurses' associations, or specialty nursing associations with local resources.

Methods of professional assistance must balance efforts to assure client/consumer welfare with a commitment to preserve the civil rights of a professional colleague. Violations of confidentiality, failure to inform nurses of their rights to legal counsel, and encouragement of the nurse to divulge self-incriminating evidence have occurred frequently in the past. Encouraging the nurse to surrender licensure in the absence of diversion legislation without identifying other options or providing consultation on the implications of this action unfairly influences a decision-making process that should be undertaken with legal counsel and a drug-free state of mind.

Efforts to control the use of illicit drugs and alcohol in the workplace must consider the civil rights of the individual. An employing institution or corporation that reserves the right to dismiss workers identified as using drugs or alcohol on or off the job must so state in their employment policies. Included in such policies should be a statement of circumstances under which body fluids of employees will be analyzed, for example, when an incident or accident occurs, or when an employee's behavior deviates from expected social or professional norms. (Nurses reentering practice after treatment for addiction generally agree to random body fluid analysis as part of the employment contract.)

Institutions that include body fluid analysis for alcohol or illicit drug use as part of preemployment screening should so state on applications for employment. In addition to stating the contingencies of employment, such policies also inform nurses seeking employment of their choice. A point of considerable concern is that findings of body fluid analysis may or may not correlate with impaired job performance. Widely used urine tests detect the metabolites of drugs; they do not measure drug intoxication at an identified period of time. Metabolites of certain drugs such as cocaine, marijuana, and barbiturates are detectable in the individual's urine for hours and often days after the use of the drug. Should a nurse returning from vacation be subject to dismissal if urinalysis indicates that marijuana has been smoked away from the site of employment as a recreational activity?

Problems of inaccuracy associated with urinalysis testing for drug use also increase the risk of unjust discipline or job termination. Urinalysis for drug use should consist of two steps: (1) screening of a sample for chemicals, and (2) confirmation tests on the split-half of the same sample to identify the presence suggested by the initial test. The most common and inexpensive screening method is immunoassay. Other screening techniques include radioimmunoassay and thin-layer chromatography.

Gas chromatography and gas chromatography/mass spectrometry (GC/MS) are considered the best confirmatory tests and are more costly than screening techniques. Some important issues regarding screening and confirmatory urinalysis include the traceability of the sample from the time it is given by the employee, through all the steps of analysis. The potential for human error is high, starting from validation by a witness that the urine sample is that of a specific employee, through secure storage and accurate test readings by the technician charged with such responsibility. Screening tests in urinalysis have reliability rates ranging from 5% to 50%. False positive findings may be reported in rates of 21% to 51% depending on the drug for which detection is conducted (Panner & Christakis, 1986). These occur for many reasons including cross-reactions between drugs and testing agents, operator errors, and the presence of endogenous substances in the urine or blood serum.

The majority of nurses employed by institutions are unaware of personal rights in relation to employment practices. Most are disinclined to question protocols and practices. The decision to utilize monitoring techniques to deter impairment of employee's performance and decisions by nursing management to support such practices pose ethical dilemmas since they may compromise the autonomy of individual nurses in the guise of beneficent practice for the consumer and employer.

The individual experiencing drug, alcohol, or psychiatric illness is bound by ethical considerations extending beyond the responsibility to seek treatment and appropriate care. The symptoms of the illness interfere with judgment and ethical decision making, and in order to access positive legal and professional sanctions, the nurse must be willing to accept the sick role inherent in addictive or psychiatric illness. For example, according to stipulations of legislation which allows a bypass of disciplinary procedures, the nurse must accept this designation in order to be granted exemption. *Diversion legislation* is so called because it diverts the individual from proceeding through the usual investigations, hearings, and state board actions which constitute the disciplinary process. The practitioner must agree to suspend the practice of nursing for the period of time specified by the agency responsible for discipline. Acknowledgment of the illness and sanctions for its appropriate treatment will not be forthcoming without the assumption of a sick role by the practitioner. Recognition of addiction as an illness, the expectation of treatment, and employment and disability benefits appropriate to quality care are rights of the professional nurse parallelled by expectations of compliance to socially acceptable behaviors.

Legal Considerations

Branches of state governments are charged to oversee the provision of quality health care to the consumer by licensed professionals. In most states, regulation of care takes the form of granting and upholding state licensure to practice. Because state governments have the right to create, interpret, and enforce laws related to licensure and practice, wide variation exists from state to state in the regulation of nursing practice.

State boards of nursing develop and conduct licensure examinations, review and make recommendations on disciplinary procedures, and study patterns of practice that relate to the distribution and function of registered nurses within the state and the nation. State board members, appointed by governing officials, have the responsibility to implement laws that promote the public welfare and protect the health care consumer.

Laws concerning impaired practice exist at state and federal levels, and new rulings are emerging in case law. Legal considerations come into play when impaired practice is suspected or identified in association with disciplinary action and when a nurse reenters practice following a period of treatment and rehabilitation. Important state laws include the state nurse practice acts, mandatory reporting laws, public health laws related to the diversion and sale of drugs, and newly passed diversion legislation.

Nurse Practice Acts

Nurse practice acts vary by state and define the practice of professional nurses in operational and legal terms. These acts are legally binding for practitioners who pass state licensure exams successfully and meet other criteria for licensure as a registered nurse. Provisions of state laws also specify conditions and acts designated as "professional misconduct." Most states list alcoholism, chronic intoxication, and drug addiction as constituting professional misconduct or incompetent practice and grounds for licensure action. Professional medical and nursing organizations have been working since the late 1960s to promote legislation and disciplinary sanctions that acknowledge addictive and psychiatric disturbances as health problems. Advocates for health professionals and organizational spokespersons argue that when "professional misconduct" is a function of these illnesses, it should be regarded as a consequence of illness rather than an intentional legal infraction. Treatment and rehabilitation are far more desirable outcomes than divestiture of the professional license, which punishes the practitioner for being ill by years of professional inactivity and economic, personal, and professional losses.

A number of state licensing boards for nursing have initiated activities to educate their members about illnesses that result in impaired practice and their appropriate treatment and rehabilitation. Through collaboration with state nurses' associations and consultation with specialty nursing organizations, they have modified disciplinary practices to reflect their primary goal, public protection, but to also support treatment, rehabilitation, and reentry of the registered nurse. State boards of nursing do not always have the ultimate power to reprimand the nurse or to suspend or revoke licensure. In New York State, for instance, final action is taken by the New York State Board of Regents after consideration of the state board's recommendations. In other states, the state attorney general criminally prosecutes the nurse based on the findings of a legal investigation. The state boards in such situations have limited power to influence established criminal process, and nursing organizations are working to produce diversion legislation to change such anachronistic and punitive processes.

In recent years legislative changes have resulted in new options for nurses whose practice has been impaired by addiction to drugs or alcohol, psychiatric illness, or senility. Diversion legislation, similar to the "sick physician's bill" passed in several states, is now being implemented in California, Florida, New York, and New Mexico. Such laws allow registered nurses and other licensed professionals to seek treatment without being subject to charges of professional misconduct. When criminal charges for theft or sale of drugs have been initiated, however, the nurse must answer to these. Programs developed from diversion legislation delineate the process by which the individual voluntarily surrenders a license if certain stipulations are met. These may include the facts that no harm has come to the client, the proposed treatment plan is acceptable to the implementing body, the nurse agrees not to practice and to notify clients of temporary withdrawal from practice, and the nurse accepts monitoring procedures as designated by the state. Such laws acknowledge that health professionals are vulnerable to illness and support rehabilitative rather than punitive action. Diversion legislation has been sanctioned by the ANA Committee on Impaired Nursing Practice as a means of providing improved health care for nurses and greater opportunities to return to practice during recovery, without the delays and lengthy process involved in reapplication for licensure.

Mandatory Reporting Laws

The mandatory reporting laws that exist in some states have direct impact on the outcomes of impaired practice cases. Where such laws are in effect, nurses in all positions, from peer to supervisor, are required to report a nurse known to them as having a drug or alcohol problem. In some instances, reporting is mandatory even though impaired job performance is not evidenced in job evaluations and when behaviors are termed "suspicious." Not only is there high potential for abuse of such legislation, but the potential for error is grave, since clinical judgement about substance abuse belongs only to experts in that field, not with supervisory personnel. Of additional concern is the absence of programs to assist nurses from the time they are reported to the time that an investigation is initiated, often a minimum of six months. Mandatory reporting that would serve to move the nurse into a state board or institutionally sponsored program could be positive in its effect of achieving early intervention. Since few states have systems or programs that function in cooperation with state nurses' associations, mandatory reporting continues to have primarily punitive results.

When impaired practice is identified and addressed in the employment setting, legal requirements influence events in at least two ways: The nurse administrator may be required by law to report an incident, including the termination or forced resignation of a nurse in relation to substance abuse, and state drug enforcement agencies may be notified and an investigation initiated. In some states, investigators of state boards of nursing are notified and become involved at the outset. Reporting of a nurse to the state board by a supervisor, peer, or consumer initiates disciplinary and possible criminal proceedings that extend over several months. During this time, the nurse is still licensed to practice unless remanded to an immediate hearing and arrest. In institutions with enlightened approaches to the problem, treatment and medical leave of absence are discussed and support services are activated through the employee assistance program and peer assistance programs. The most negative outcomes are the firing or the forced resignation of the nurse, because they result in the loss of the individual to the employing agency and the loss of opportunities to move the nurse into treatment. Drug enforcement agencies and the state department of health may further initiate criminal charges, which result in investigations and fines, distinct from disciplinary outcomes.

Legal Rights of the Nurse

When an investigation or confrontation occurs in the workplace, many nurses are unaware of the right to engage legal counsel and the importance of doing so. Often, diversion of drugs from hospital supplies precipitates the event. The nurse's befogged mental state and the involvement of hospital security or police, hospital administrators and nursing supervisors all create a powerful scenario which often evokes compliance to treatment on the nurse's part. At the same time, the nurse's rights to the presence of a supportive family member and legal counsel are often ignored. When attempts to obtain a "confession" or provide self-incriminating evidence are initiated by drug enforcement officials or state board investigators, the nurse's civil rights are similarly violated. Such efforts, which become the basis of legal charges, obscure the goals of motivating the nurse to seek treatment and rehabilitation.

In employment settings where state nurses' associations maintain collective bargaining units, assistance supported by state law also takes the form of union action. Grievance committees and union representatives can help the nurse gain access to health care benefits, including medical leave and disability. Members of economic and general welfare committees act as advocates for the nurse within the system, provide testimony, and negotiate with management about plans for treatment and reentry. The support of colleagues knowledgeable about employment practices and resources has been a key in initiating treatment for large numbers of nurses.

Reentry to Practice

Federal and state laws are particularly relevant as the nurse prepares to reenter practice. Decisions about the readiness to return to practice are made by the nurse with the treatment agency or care provider. Peer support groups and self-help, 12-step programs (like Alcoholics Anonymous or Narcotics Anonymous) also provide important resources. If action has been taken on the nurse's license by state regulatory agencies, the conditions of probation or suspension must be successfully met before the nurse can consider reentry. If licensure has been revoked, the reapplication process must be initiated and completed. In some states, legal requirements include a monitoring system organized by the state board for nursing or other monitoring systems for health professionals such as those through employee assistance programs.

Application for employment and the return to professional life is facilitated by the fact that federal legislation requires that records of a treatment facility receiving any amount of federal funding be confidential. They are not accessible without the permission of the individual treated. This requirement applies even when reentry contracts are in effect, and the agency or employee assistance program accepts responsibility for monitoring the nurse's continuation of treatment. Concerns about revealing information are real and important, and recovering nurses as well as their advocates should be informed of legal rights in this regard.

Federal legislation relevant to return to work has also been passed. Section 504 of the Federal Rehabilitation Act (1973), which prohibits discrimination against the handicapped, addresses the issue of alcohol and drug abuse as handicaps. States may or may not acknowledge federal legislation but at least 35 states have laws prohibiting discrimination against the handicapped and several cases have upheld the applicability of the federal act. Sections of the act that relate to employment exclude the active alcoholic or drug abuser whose employment could constitute a threat to the safety or property of others. The act has several relevant provisions, however, for the recovering nurse returning to employment, since it prohibits discrimination in hiring when nurses have histories of addiction to alcohol and have successfully undergone treatment. Federal legislation is less frequently interpreted to apply to recovering drug addicts, although many states recognize addiction to drugs as a handicap.

The Federal Rehabilitation Act states that the employer has the responsibility to provide reasonable modifications in the work place to accommodate the handicapped individual. For the returning nurse, such accommodations may include employment on units where controlled substances are rarely utilized, stable shift assignments, or office employment where medications are stocked in limited numbers. Several cases in which the rehabilitation act has been favorably interpreted for the recovering individual are on record, and this legislation is an important resource.

As the health professions acquire knowledge about the nature and effective treatment of illnesses that result in impairment, policy and position statements will be increasingly valuable reference points. Impairment is an issue of importance to nursing and its professional advancement, and nursing must respond to responsibilities to its members and the consumer. Support of the individual practitioner of nursing also advances efforts to contain the problem. Support is increased by quality health care benefits and a safe working environment where medications are adequately controlled. Consultation and assistance with stress management and education on substance abuse are key supports that further the professions's efforts to contain the problem and prevent it in the future.

References

American Nurses Association (1976). *Code for Nurses with interpretative statements.* Kansas City, MO: Author.

American Nurses' Association. (1984). M. Naegle (Ed.), *Addictions and psychological dysfunctions: The profession's response to the problem.* Kansas City, MO.

Morrow, C. K. (1984). Doctors helping doctors. *The Hastings Center Report.* December, 32–38.

Naegle, M. (1985). Creative management of impaired nursing practice. *Nursing Administration Quarterly,* 9(3), 16–26.

Panner, M., and A. Christakis. (1986). The limits of science in on-the-job screening. *The Hastings Center Report.* December, 8, 7–12.

Rosen, T. (1987). Detection of substance abuse in the work place: One consultant's perspective. Unpublished paper.

Spencer, J. M. (1979). The developing notion of employer responsibility for the alcoholic, drug addicted or mentally ill employee. *St. John's Law Review,* (53)4, 660–720.

2

Attitudes Toward Chemically Dependent Nurses: Care or Curse?

Tonda L. Hughes and Eleanor J. Sullivan

Attitudes toward chemical dependency in both society and nursing are among the most important factors thought to influence institutional and professional responses to nurses impaired by the use or abuse of chemical substances. Like the general public, many health professionals question whether or not chemical dependency is a disease when personal choice seems so clearly to play a role in its development. Such attitudes act as barriers to identification, intervention, referral, rehabilitation, and reentry into the professional work setting. They also work against the establishment of uniform, systematic, and humane policies for dealing with the chemically dependent nurses.

Historical Background

Views of chemical dependency have varied markedly across time as well as across social and cultural groups. During the last two hundred years alcoholism has alternately been viewed as a problem of the "will" or as an "illness" or "disease" (Orcutt, Cairl, & Miller,

1980). The view that habitual drinking is a form of illness is not new. In fact, Benjamin Rush, an eminent American physician of the 18th century, wrote that drunkenness ". . . resembles certain hereditary, family and contagious diseases" (Rush, reprinted 1943). Throughout the 19th century, the concept that alcoholism is a disease continued to hold a central place in the writings of researchers interested in alcoholism.

In the United States, this view lost considerable credibility during the prohibition era (1920–1933). Although the disease concept was revived shortly thereafter, first by Alcoholics Anonymous and later through the work of Jellinek (1960), the moral view has generally held sway despite strenuous efforts by some professional organizations to counter it (Orcutt, 1976; Tournier, 1985). For example, the American Medical Association passed a resolution in 1956 urging hospitals to admit patients diagnosed as having alcoholism as they would admit patients with other diagnoses (JAMA, 1956).

Views of drug addiction have also changed over time. Opium and its derivatives were openly used in this country for a wide variety of human ills until the early 20th century and, in fact, were considered by many less offensive than cigarette smoking (Clausen, 1977). It is estimated that there were 200,000 narcotic addicts in the United States in 1924, two-thirds of whom were women (Terry & Pellens cited in Ogur, 1986). Addiction was treated as a legitimate medical problem until the passage of the Harrison Narcotic Act in 1914; subsequently, the addict was defined as a criminal and branded a "dope fiend, degenerate, and enemy of society." This shift in perspective served to increase greatly the difficulty of rehabilitating addicts and assimilating them into mainstream society (Clausen, 1977, p. 27). Only recently has the public returned to the belief that drug addiction is to some extent a treatable illness (Pattison, Bishop, & Linsky, 1968).

At present, an increased acceptance of the disease concept has mitigated somewhat the stigma of chemical dependency and thus increased the number of people willing to seek treatment. However, studies indicate that moralistic views of alcoholism and drug addiction are still widely held (Dean & Poremba, 1983; Dean & Rud, 1984; Tournier, 1985). Often these seemingly disparate attitudes coexist within the same individual (Mulford & Miller, 1964; Orcutt, 1976; Tournier, 1985).

Perceptions of chemical dependency are important because the way a problem is defined influences the selection of a particular therapeutic strategy (Caplan & Nelson, 1973). For example, both Stoll (1968) and Parsons (1964) have suggested that methods of controlling deviants follow from assumptions about the causes of the deviant behaviors. Pattison, Bishop, and Linsky (1968) summarize the position as follows:

> If the individual himself is seen as the causal agent and as able to control his behavior he is held responsible and morally blamable, and society supports punitive responses with little concern for rehabilitation. If, however, the causal agent is seen as external factors, the individual is assumed to have little control over his behavior, is not held responsible or morally blamable, and society supports rehabilitative measures. (p. 160)

This position is supported in studies on attitudes toward alcoholics and drug addicts (Mogar et al., 1969; Pattison et al., 1968; Reisman & Shrader, 1984; Romney & Bynner, 1985). For example, Mulford and Miller (1964) found that people who viewed alcoholism as an illness were more in favor of therapeutic intervention than were those who viewed the alcoholic as morally weak. When studying the relationship between occupational health nurses' attitudes toward alcoholics and treatment referral rates, Reisman and Shrader (1984) discovered that nurses who held the more "positive" attitude that alcoholism is a treatable illness were more likely to make referrals than those nurses whose attitudes were less favorable.

Attitudes of Health Professionals

The influence of health professionals' attitudes on their response to and care of chemically dependent clients has long been a topic of concern. For example, physicians' general unwillingness to identify and manage alcoholic patients is amply documented (Chafetz, 1968; Fisher, Keeley, Mason, & Fisher, 1975; Hanna, 1978; Rathod, 1967; Sterne & Pittman, 1965; Wolf, Chafetz, Blane, & Hill, 1968).

Allen, Peterson, and Keating (1982) conducted a study of 40 mental health and rehabilitation counselors. These counselors were found to hold significantly more negative attitudes toward alcoholics than toward homosexuals, public offenders, the mentally retarded, the physically disabled, and the mentally ill.

In a study conducted by Sterne and Pittman (1965), nurses were found to be considerably more moralistic regarding alcoholism than were physicians or social workers. Subsequent studies conducted in the 1960s and 1970s have added considerable support to the finding that nurses generally hold negative attitudes (e.g., moral weakness as the cause and punitive treatment for the cure) toward alcoholics (Chodorkoff, 1969; Cornish & Miller, 1976; Ferneau & Morton, 1968; Moody, 1971; Schmid & Schmid, 1973; Wallston, Wallston, & DeVellis, 1976).

Fewer studies have been done on attitudes of health professionals toward drug addicts and drug addiction; fewer still have examined nurses' attitudes. Sowa and Cutter (1974) explored the attitudes of various hospital staff toward alcoholics and drug addicts. These investigators found that nurses tend to hold more positive attitudes about alcoholics and drug addicts than do psychologists and psychiatrists, and that nurses (as well as other staff) hold more favorable attitudes toward alcoholics than toward drug addicts. Conversely, a study of Nevada nurses found that nurses, as compared to other professional groups, were less optimistic, more moralistic, and more inclined to stereotype substance abusers (Veach, 1987).

Recent studies by Engs (1982) and Sullivan and Hale (1987), however, indicate that nurses' attitudes (at least toward alcoholics) may now be more positive than those reflected in previous studies. Using Tolor and Tamerin's (1975) Attitudes Toward Alcoholism Questionnaire, Sullivan and Hale (1987) surveyed a national sample of 1,026 registered nurses. Respondents reported strong support for the belief that alcoholism has either a psychological or physical/genetic cause and that alcoholics should receive therapeutic medical care. There was little support for moral weakness as a causative factor in alcoholism. Respondents' beliefs did not differ based on the nurses' age, length of time in nursing practice, clinical specialty area, position, or employment setting. Using the same instrument as did Sullivan and Hale, Engs (1982) found nursing students' attitudes to be more positive (i.e., more support for physical or psychological versus moral weakness as the cause) than students in other health professions.

The Influence of Education on Attitudes

The effect of education about alcoholism and drug addiction on professionals' attitudes toward alcoholics and drug addicts has also been explored in some depth (Cartwright, 1980; Finke, 1986; Kinney, Price, & Bergen, 1984; Long, 1986; Waring, 1975). The lack of accurate information about chemical dependency is thought to be closely related to attitudes toward such behavior. That is, lack of understanding of the addictive process is thought to perpetuate and reinforce stereotypical views of alcoholics and drug addicts (Harlow & Goby, 1980).

Studies in the literature report conflicting outcomes of educational programs aimed at changing attitudes. For example, both Harlow and Goby (1980) and Long (1986) report improved attitudes toward alcoholism (i.e., more accepting and less judgmental) in students who participated in alcoholism educational programs. However, other studies have found little or no change in attitudes following participation in alcoholism educational programs (e.g., Waring, 1975) or improved attitudes toward alcoholics and drug addicts generally, but no change in attitudes toward the alcoholic or drug-addicted nurse (LaBrosse, 1987).

Historically, nurses have received little content in their educational curricula regarding the addictive process (Burkhalter, 1975; Burton, 1971; Carter, 1983; Einstein & Wolfson, 1970; Gurel, 1974; Hoffman & Heinemann, 1987). When content on alcoholism and drug addiction is included, such information generally has focused on the physiologic and toxic effects of alcohol and other drugs and has included little that would aid nurses in understanding the psychologic process of addiction.

In the last 10 to 15 years, efforts to improve health professionals' understanding of addiction have increased. Some progress has been made not only in developing specialized programs (Chappel, Veach, & Krug, 1984; Heinemann, 1986), but also in adding content to preexisting programs, particularly in nursing and medicine (Clark, Kachoyeanos, & Solari-Twadell, 1987; Evan & Whaite, 1982; Lewis, Niven, Czechowicz, & Trumble, 1987). For example, the University of Washington School of Nursing established the first specialized program to prepare nurses in the field of alcoholism. More recently, programs for nurses who wish to specialize in chemical dependency have been developed at the University of Maryland and the Medical College of Georgia. While considerably more programs have been developed in medical schools than in nursing schools, the most well-known are those at Brown University and Dartmouth College.

The Effect of Attitudes on Professional Response to Impairment

While attitudes toward chemical dependency have generally begun to shift from a punitive to a more rehabilitative view, this latter view is less likely when the chemically dependent person is a health care professional (LaBrosse, 1987). For example, a statewide survey of perceptions of and attitudes toward nurse impairment showed that nurses are more likely to view nurse impairment as an illness when it involves emotional distress than when it is caused by alcohol abuse. Similarly, nurse respondents reported stronger support of disciplinary measures for impairment resulting from alcohol or drug abuse than for impaired functioning caused by emotional distress (Hendrix, Sabritt, McDaniel, & Field, 1987).

Not only do professional ethics dictate that nurses intervene whenever consumer safety is at risk, but concern for colleagues requires nurses to intervene when chemical impairment is suspected. However, despite the growing recognition that nurses are practicing while chemically impaired, denial of such problems continues.

It is widely reported in the literature that chemically impaired nurses are rarely confronted or are confronted only after the situation is no longer possible to ignore (Bissell & Jones, 1981; Hughes, 1987; Isler, 1978; Jaffe, 1982; Naegle, 1985; O'Connor & Robinson, 1985; Patrick, 1984).

Stereotypic and stigmatic attitudes toward alcoholism and drug addiction contribute both directly and indirectly to the lack of response to chemical dependency in colleagues. Chemically dependent nurses do not fit the commonly held image of an alcoholic or drug addict, and coworkers can easily attribute signs and symptoms of a progressing addiction to the impaired colleague's stressful work or home environment. Furthermore, even when chemical dependency is strongly suspected, nurses are reluctant to report their suspicions, since in most cases such information will lead to termination of employment and in many instances, professional and legal sanctions. While failure to intervene may reflect a desire to protect a colleague from these punitive sanctions, such "enabling" responses deny the chemically impaired nurse much needed assistance and place at continued risk those patients for whom the nurse is responsible.

The influence of attitudes extends beyond the individual and is demonstrated by the lack of formal guidelines for dealing with chemical dependency among nurses. Currently, relatively few hospitals and other health care facilities have clearly articulated policies and procedures governing response to nurses whose functioning is compromised by the use or abuse of chemical substances (Chaney, 1987; Hughes, 1986, 1988). Thus, chemical dependency is indirectly perpetuated by management's reluctance to confront the nature of nurses' performance problems. When forced to respond, management commonly requests the nurse's resignation or automatically dismisses the nurse.

As evidenced in a study of documents related to State Board criteria for licensure and disciplinary procedures, a lack of guidelines also exists at the state regulatory level (Champagne, Havens, & Swenson, 1987). These investigators note that while "habitual intemperance, addiction to habit-forming drugs, or the use of such substances to the extent that they interfere with competent care" (p. 56) are consistently identified as conditions warranting disciplinary action, what form that action might take is not made explicit. They further note that few statements related to care, counseling, or other rehabilitative measures were found in the documents analyzed (p. 57).

A number of states have laws that mandate reporting nurses who are suspected of being chemically dependent. In the absence of policies and procedures that would assist the nurse into treatment and facilitate reentry into the workforce following treatment, such laws act primarily as "policing" tactics that punish chemically dependent nurses and, ironically, do more to deter than to facilitate reporting.

Attitudes Toward Chemically Dependent Women

Attitudes toward chemically dependent nurses cannot be separated from attitudes toward chemically dependent women. It is a well accepted dictum that alcoholic and drug-addicted women are more harshly stigmatized than are alcoholic and drug-addicted men. For women who are nurses, the stigma of chemical dependency is likely magnified. Thus, one reason for the reluctance of management to deal openly with chemical dependency among nursing staff is likely related to the fact that nursing has been and continues to be a predominately female profession.

Although readily acknowledged as essential to the day-to-day operation of most health care institutions, nurses generally are not paid commensurate with their level of responsibility. Nurses tend to be more valued for their caretaking and nurturing roles than for their education and training, which enable them to perform multiple and often complex roles within a diverse range of health care settings.

Physicians, because they are often self employed and work relatively unsupervised, are less likely to be terminated from employment or lose their license for chemical dependency. For physicians who do have problems with their jobs or licenses, more resources are available. Not only do physicians have more financial resources for legal fees and treatment, there are currently physician's assistance programs in every state. These programs provide a variety of services including intervention, referral, and financial assistance. Chemically dependent nurses, on the other hand, because they are generally less valued employees and because of the nature of their work situations have been regularly subject to termination, to arrest and prosecution, as well as to prolonged or permanent loss of license.

One example of the differential treatment of physicians and nurses was a recent highly publicized arrest of nurses in the Chicago, Illinois area. Following are excerpts from news releases broadcast on leading Chicago television stations:

> State police have begun an arrest roundup of sixteen registered nurses, most of them from the Chicago area, on charges of illegal drug use. The

> arrest began at six A.M. this morning. Those taken into custody were taken to various police lockups, including this state police post . . . (Eyewitness News, 1986)
>
> . . . authorities claim the sixteen nurses acting individually used a variety of techniques to get their hands on drugs intended for patients. They stole from hospital carts; they forged doctors' signatures on prescriptions; they ordered medication for patients who had already died. And they used one more technique that endangered the patients themselves: In some cases, nurses would take containers of the painkiller Demerol,® load up the syringe as if to give it to the patient, then inject herself. To cover up the theft, she would reload the container with water or saline solution, so the patient ended up getting an injection of water instead of pain killer (Channel 2 News at Five, 1986).

While this roundup of nurses was reportedly "just the start of a crackdown on the problem of drug diversion by doctors and nurses," the arrests followed a six-month investigation by state regulatory officials and occurred more than a year after mandatory reporting requirement amendments to the Illinois Nursing Act took effect. Furthermore, while almost every media report of the arrests hinted that physicians would be targeted next, if physicians were arrested, those arrests were not made public.

Professional Response

It is finally becoming more widely recognized and accepted that while protection of the consumer is an important and legitimate concern, this concern should not preclude supportive responses to the chemically dependent nurse.

The earliest efforts to ameliorate the problems of impaired practice were begun in the 1970s by nurses recovering from alcohol and/or drug dependency. These nurses, painfully aware of the stigma associated with impairment and lack of resources to deal with it, started grassroots programs to educate the profession about chemical dependence.

The first attempt to pass a resolution at the national level concerning impaired practice failed in 1980. However, in 1982, the ANA

House of Delegates, recognizing its responsibility to the public, to nurses, and to the profession, formally acknowledged and took action on the issue of impaired functioning caused by drugs, alcohol, or psychological dysfunction. The resolution calls for development of guidelines for assistance programs, the encouragement of nursing administrators and other employers of nurses to offer appropriate services *prior* to disciplinary action, and the establishment of mechanisms to collect and disseminate information related to the issue of impairment (ANA, 1982).

At this time, special committees and peer assistance programs have been developed, or are in process of being developed, in many states to address the issue of impaired practice. The primary goal of these programs is to identify the impaired nurse and to facilitate entry into treatment. Therefore, considerable efforts have focused on educating staff in hospitals and other health care institutions about the importance and appropriateness of intervening whenever chemical dependency is suspected.

In addition, a number of professional nursing organizations, including the ANA Task Force on Addictions and Psychological Dysfunctions, the National Nurses Society on Addictions, and the Drug and Alcohol Nurses Association, as well as committees and groups in various states, are actively working to modify current disciplinary practices and to encourage the adoption of uniform policies and laws that support intervention and treatment, rather than termination and prosecution.

Conclusion

Chemical use behaviors influence and are influenced by cultural attitude sets in the home, in schools, among professional groups, and in society generally. These attitudes can either assist or hinder interventions into the problem of chemical use and dependency among various subgroups of the population. Because attitudes of the general public and nurses themselves toward impairment may still be somewhat punitive rather than rehabilitative, it is important that the profession fully acknowledge the problem and formulate standards and guidelines to ameliorate its effects.

If we, as health professionals, view chemical dependency in others as a tragic and treatable illness, can we legitimately accord less care and compassion to members of our own profession? Can we justify treating one group of people while punishing members of another?

It is hoped that as nurses and other health professionals gain knowledge about the nature and effective treatment of addictive illness, policies demonstrating compassion, understanding, and caring for the nurse, as well as concern for the well-being of the client, the profession, and the health care institution will be the rule rather than the exception.

References

Allen, H. A., Peterson, J. S., & Keating, G. (1982). Attitudes of counselors toward the alcoholic. *Rehabilitation Counseling Bulletin, January,* 162–164.

American Nurses' Association House of Delegates. (1982). *Action on alcohol and drug misuse and psychological dysfunctions among nurses.* Resolution #5, adopted June 29, 1982.

Bissell, L., & Jones, R. W. (1981). The alcoholic nurse. *Nursing Outlook, 29*(2), 96–101.

Burkhalter, P. (1975). Alcoholism, drug abuse and drug addiction: A study of nursing education. *Journal of Nursing Education, 14*(2), 30–36.

Burton, G. (1971). Nursing education on alcoholism. *Annals of the New York Academy of Science, 178,* 48–51.

Caplan, N., & Nelson, S. D. (1973). On being useful. The nature and consequences of psychological research on social problems. *American Psychologist, 28,* 199–211.

Carter, A. J. (1983). Nurses: Alcohol and drug abuse training in nursing schools. *Alcohol Health and Research World, 8,* 24–29.

Cartright, A. K. J. (1980). The attitudes of helping agents toward the alcoholic client: The influence of experience, support, training and self-esteem. *British Journal of the Addictions, 75*(4), 413–431.

Chafetz, M. E. (1968). Research in the alcohol clinic and around-the-clock psychiatric service of the Massachusetts General Hospital. *American Journal of Psychiatry, 124,* 1674–1679.

Champagne, M., Havens, B., & Swenson, I. (1987). State board criteria for licensure and disciplinary procedures regarding impaired nurses. *Nursing Outlook, 35*(2), 54–57, 101.

Chaney, E. A. (1987). Nurses and chemical dependency: Policy considerations. *Journal of Pediatric Nursing, 2*(1), 61–63.

Channel 2 News at Five. (1987, February 28). Transcript of WBBM-TV (CBS) news report.

Chappel, J., Veach, T. L., & Krug, R. S. (1984). The substance abuse attitude survey: An instrument for measuring attitudes. *Journal of Studies on Alcohol, 46*(1), 48–52.

Chodorkoff, B. (1969). Alcoholism education in a psychiatric institute. II. Student nurses, relationship of personal characteristics, attitudes toward alcoholism and achievement. *Quarterly Journal of Studies on Alcoholism, 30,* 657–664.

Clark, M. D., Kachoyeanos, M., & Solari-Twadell, A. (1987). Educating the educators on alcoholism. *Nursing Success Today, 3*(17), 21–23.

Clausen, J. A. (1977). Early history of narcotics use and narcotics legislation in the United States. In P. E. Rock (Ed.), *Drugs and Politics* (pp. 23–29). New Brunswick, NJ: Transaction Books.

Cornish, R. D., & Miller, M. V. (1976). Attitudes of registered nurses toward the alcoholic. *Journal of Psychiatric Nursing and Mental Health Services, 14*(2), 19–22.

Dean, J. C., & Poremba, G. A. (1983). The alcoholic stigma and the disease concept. *The International Journal of the Addictions, 18,* 739–751.

Dean, J. C., & Rud, F. (1984). The drug addict and the stigma of addiction. *The International Journal of the Addictions, 19,* 859–869.

Einstein, S., & Wolfson, E. (1970). Alcoholism curriculum: How professionals are trained. *International Journal of the Addictions, 5*(2), 295–312.

Engs, R. (1982). Medical, nursing and pharmacy students' attitudes toward alcoholism in Queensland, Australia. *Alcoholism: Clinical and Experimental Research, 6*(2), 225–229.

Evan, C. E., & Whaite, A. (1982). Training health professionals in substance abuse: A review. *The International Journal of the Addictions, 17*(7), 1211–1229.

Eyewitness News. (1986, February, 28). Transcript of WLS-TV (ABC) news report.

Ferneau, E. W., & Morton, E. L. (1968). Nursing personnel and alcoholism. *Nursing Research, 17,* 174–177.

Finke, L. M. (1986). Effect of an educational program on the role of security of medical-surgical nurses towards confronting clients with drinking problems. *Dissertation Abstracts International, 46*(10), 3390B–3391B (University Microfilms No. DA8526792).

Fisher, J. C., Keeley, K. A., Mason, R. L., & Fisher, J. V. (1975). Physicians and alcoholics: Factors affecting attitudes of family practice residents toward alcoholics. *Journal of Studies on Alcohol, 36,* 626–633.

Gurel, M. (1974). Should courses for nurses that deal solely with alcoholism be taught in universities? *Nursing Research, 23*(2), 166–169.

Hanna, E. (1978). Attitudes toward problem drinkers. *Journal of Studies on Alcohol, 1,* 98–109.

Harlow, P. E., & Goby, M. J. (1980). Changing nursing students' attitudes toward alcoholic patients: Examining effects of a clinical practicum. *Nursing Research, 29*(1), 59–60.

Heinemann, E. (1986). *Substance abuse in schools of nursing: A national survey.* Presentation at the First National Impaired Nurse Symposium and Research Conference, Atlanta, GA.

Hendrix, M. J., Sabritt, D., McDaniel, A., & Field, B. (1987). Perceptions and attitudes toward nursing impairment. *Research in Nursing and Health, 10,* 323–333.

Hoffman, A. L., & Heinemann, M. E. (1987). Substance abuse education in schools of nursing: A national survey. *Journal of Nursing Education, 26*(7), 282–287.

Hughes, T. L. (1986). *Chemical impairment in nursing: Attitudes and perceptions of first-level nursing administrators.* Unpublished manuscript.

Hughes, T. L. (1987). Chemical impairment in nursing. *Nursing RSA Verpleging* (Scientific Journal of the South African Nursing Association), *2* (4), 5–7, 9,40.

Hughes, T. L. (1988, March). *Chief nurse executives' responses to chemically dependent nurses: The influence of institutional, personal, and contextual factors.* Presentation at the Sixth National Impaired Nurse Symposium and Research Conference, Atlanta, GA.

Isler, C. (1978). The alcoholic nurse: What we try to deny. *RN, 41*(7), 48–55.

Jaffe, S. (1982). Help for the helper: First hand views of recovery. *American Journal of Nursing, 82*(5), 578–579.

Jellinek, E. M. (1960). *The disease concept of alcoholism.* New Haven, CT: Hillhouse.

Journal of the American Medical Association. (1956). (Reports of Officers). Hospitalization of patients with alcoholism. *Journal of the American Medical Association, 162,* 750.

Kinney, J., Price, T. R. P., & Bergen, B. J. (1984). Impediments to alcohol education. *Journal of Studies on Alcohol, 45*(5), 453–459.

LaBrosse, P. A. (1987). *The effect of an educational program on attitudes of nursing students toward chemical dependency.* Presentation at the Fifth National Impaired Nurse Symposium and Research Conference, Atlanta, GA.

Lewis, D. C., Niven, R. G., Czechowicz, E., & Trumble, J. G. (1987). A review of medical education in alcoholism and drug abuse. *Journal of the American Medical Association, 257*(21), 2945–2948.

Long, P. (1986). Effect of an alcoholism education program on student nurses' attitudes toward alcoholism. *Dissertation Abstracts International, 46*(12), 3610A. (University Microfilms No. DA8526102).

Mogar, R. E., Helm, S. T., Snedeker, M. R., Snedeker, M. H., & Wilson, W. M. (1969). Staff attitudes toward the alcoholic patient. *Archives of General Psychiatry, 21,* 449–454.

Moody, P. M. (1971). Attitudes of nurses and nursing students toward alcoholism treatment. *Quarterly Journal of Studies on Alcohol, 32,* 172–175.

Mulford, H. A., & Miller, D. E. (1964). Public acceptance of the alcoholic as sick. *Quarterly Journal of Studies on Alcohol, 25,* 314–324.

Naegle, M. A. (1985). Creative management of impaired nursing practice. *Nursing Administration Quarterly, 9*(3), 16–26.

O'Connor, P., & Robinson, R. S. (1985). Managing impaired nurses. *Nursing Administration Quarterly, 9*(2), 1–9.

Ogur, B. (1986). Long day's journey into night: Women and prescription drug abuse. *Women and Health, 11*(1), 99–115.

Orcutt, J. D. (1976). Ideological variations in the structure of deviant types: A multivariate comparison of alcoholism and heroin addiction. *Social Forces, 55,* 419–437.

Orcutt, J. D., Cairl, R. E., & Miller, E. T. (1980). Professional and public conceptions of alcoholism. *Journal of Studies on Alcohol, 41*(7), 652–661.

Parsons, T. (1964). *Social structure and personality.* New York: The Free Press.

Patrick, P. K. S. (1984). Self-preservation: Confronting the issue of nurse impairment. *Journal of Substance Abuse Treatment, 1*(2), 99–105.

Pattison, E. M., Bishop, L. A., & Linsky, A. S. (1968). Changes in public attitudes on narcotic addiction. *American Journal of Psychiatry, 125,* 160–167.

Rathod, N. H. (1967). An inquiry into general practitioners' opinions about alcoholism. *British Journal of Addictions, 62,* 103–111.

Reisman, B. L., & Shrader, R. W. (1984). Effect of nurses' attitudes toward alcoholics on their referral rate for treatment. *Occupational Health Nursing, 32*(5), 273–275.

Romney, D. M., & Bynner, J. (1985). Hospital staff's perceptions of the alcoholic. *The International Journal of the Addictions, 20,* 393–402.

Rush, B. (1943/original 1785). An inquiry into the effects of ardent spirits upon the human body and mind, with an account of the means of preventing and of the remedies for curing them. (Reprint) *Quarterly Journal of Studies on Alcohol, 4,* 324–341.

Schmid, N. J., & Schmid, D. T. (1973). Nursing students' attitudes toward alcoholics. *Nursing Research, 22*(3), 246–248.

Sowa, P. A., & Cutter, H. S. (1974). Attitudes of hospital staff toward alcoholics and drug addicts. *Quarterly Journal of Studies on Alcohol, 35,* 210–214.

Sterne, M., & Pittman, D. (1965). The concept of motivation: A source of institutional and professional blockage in the treatment of alcoholics. *Quarterly Journal of Studies on Alcohol, 26,* 41–57.

Stoll, C. S. (1968). Images of man and social control. *Social Forces, 47,* 119–127.

Sullivan, E. J., & Hale, R. E. (1987). Nurses' beliefs about the etiology and treatment of alcohol abuse. *Journal of Studies on Alcohol, 48*(5), 456–460.

Tolar A., & Tamerin, J. S. (1975). The attitudes toward alcoholism instrument: A measure of attitudes toward alcoholics and the nature and causes of alcoholism. *British Journal of Addictions, 70,* 223–231.

Tournier, R. E. (1985). The medicalization of alcoholism: Discontinuities in ideologies of deviance. *Journal of Drug Issues, 15,* 39–49.

Veach, C. (1987). *Nevada nurses' attitudes toward substance abuse.* Presentation at the Fifth National Impaired Nurse Symposium and Research Conference, Atlanta, GA.

Wallston, K. A., Wallston, B. S., & DeVellis, B. M. (1976). Effect of a negative stereotype on nurses' attitudes toward an alcoholic patient. *Journal of Studies on Alcohol, 37*(5), 659–665.

Waring, M. L. (1975). The impact of specialized training in alcoholism on management-level professionals. *Journal of Studies on Alcohol, 36*(3), 406–415.

Wolf, I., Chafetz, M. E., Blane, H. T., & Hill, M. J. (1965). Social factors in the diagnosis of alcoholism. II. Attitudes of physicians. *Quarterly Journal of Studies on Alcohol, 26,* 72–79.

3

Community-Based Programs: Two California Models for Intervention

Marty Jessup and Jean Sullivan

Community-based programs in California emanated from an awareness of the serious problem of chemical dependency in the nursing profession and a desire to "help the helper." The Bay Area Task Force for Impaired Nurses (BATFIN)* in San Francisco and DISCOVERY** in Los Angeles are two such model programs that were established to provide a broad spectrum of intervention, consultation, and peer support services to the drug and alcohol dependent nurse, as well as legal and other referrals. These programs, both founded in the early 1980s, focused on treatment oriented intervention in the workplace, education of nurses and hospital administrators, and the use of positive peer role modeling as methods to assist nurses with chemical dependency. The central goals of both

*The Bay Area Task Force for Impaired Nurses, a time-limited grant project, was founded by Marty Jessup and Millicent Buxton in the spring of 1981 in San Francisco. Ms. Jessup would like to thank Ms. Buxton, the California Nurses Association, the Haight Ashbury Free Medical Clinic, and Dr. David E. Smith for their support.

**DISCOVERY was established by Jean Sullivan and Meredith Hardy, a licensed Clinical Social Worker, in Los Angeles in the Summer of 1983. The authors would like to thank Ms. Hardy for providing the information for the legal issues section of this chapter; since 1984, she has been an attorney practicing in California.

programs were to facilitate the nurse's treatment and to provide support when the recovering nurse returned to nursing practice. With respect to DISCOVERY, a treatment component has also been a part of the program as described below.

Scope of the Problem: Early Research

There are 250,000 nurses in the state of California. Using the statistics from studies done on the general population which indicate the incidence of chemical dependency to be 10%, we have estimated there are 25,000 chemically dependent nurses in California. During the first six months of 1980, 67% of the license probations actions by the California Board of Registered Nursing (BRN) were drug related; 87% of the license revocations were a result of licensee chemical dependency problems (Board of Registered Nursing, State of California, personal communication, 1981).

Concerned about the reliability of mortality statistics for the addicted nurse, BATFIN in 1981 examined death certificates of nurses in the city and county of San Francisco. They found that during the period of January 1, 1980 through July 1, 1983, 39 nurses died from complications associated with alcoholism and/or other drug dependency. The average age of these nurses at the time of death was 31 years. In effect, one nurse was dying every five weeks in San Francisco alone as a result of an addictive disease (Buxton, Jessup, & Landry, 1985).

In 1983 BATFIN described a profile of the chemically dependent nurse and collected demographic data on 25 nurses who requested assistance from BATFIN's support group. Each of the nurses in this group had completed at least six months recovery from alcoholism and/or other drug addiction; each completed a ten-page questionnaire. Relevant results from this study are shown in Table 3.1. It is interesting to note here that in this BATFIN sample, 16 of the nurses reported that they had at least one chemically dependent parent; and nurses who reported that both parents were addicted also tended to report that their own addictive process began at an earlier age (Buxton & Jessup, 1983).

Hardy (1983) conducted a study of anonymous case files from the California Department of Justice, Licensing Section in Los Angeles.

During the period from January 1, 1982 through June 30, 1983, 101 disciplinary proceedings were initiated against registered nurses in Los Angeles County. Of these, 97% were for drug diversion by the registered nurse. From this 97%, a random sample of 22 case files were chosen for the study. In 50% of the 22, information regarding stress factors was found. Of these, 64% indicated family/marital problems, 18% depression, 18% overwork, and 18% physical complaints. The total is over 100% since some nurses indicate more than one stressor. Further, in 67% of the sample, file information included the stated purpose for the diversion by the nurse: 100% indicated self-administration (including two who were also diverting for seriously ill family members). Other relevant results of this study are shown in Table 3.1.

Lastly, DISCOVERY compiled demographic information from the responses of 103 nurses who had sought initial assessment interviews at that program (Sullivan, 1986). Results of this study are also shown in Table 3.1. The reader is reminded that these studies were done independently, not with the purpose of coordinating these findings. However, a beginning profile of the chemically dependent nurse has emerged from these studies and from the experience of the staffs of these programs. As indicated in the table, all three studies show Demerol® to be the most commonly diverted drug, because it is the most available and most commonly used. It is also interesting to note the high percentage of critical care nurses represented in all three studies. This may be due to the high stress level, as well as the frequent losses critical care nurses experience as patients die. Nurses, traditionally, have not been taught to deal with death and loss through a healthy grieving process. The studies do suggest these and other areas where further investigation might be useful, as discussed later in this chapter.

Initial Assessment

Assessment of the nurse seeking help from one of the community-based programs described here usually occurred in an office setting where anonymity and confidentiality were preserved. The session consisted of an individual interview during which the nurse's history

TABLE 3.1 A Profile of the Chemically Dependent Nurse: Three Research Studies

Study	N	Percentage M	Percentage F	Avg. age	Years in field	Percentage in crit. care	Percentage Demerol	Percentage Other drugs
BATFIN (1983)	25	36	64	38.3	3[a]	57	95	16
Hardy (1983)	22	4	96	34.0	7.2[b]	41	91	—
Sullivan (1986)	103	23.5	76.5	36.0	9.2[c]	41	65	2

[a]Prior to first administration.
[b]Prior to incident resulting in administrative action.
[c]Prior to first contact with DISCOVERY.

was taken and the level of the nurse's denial and the degree of motivation for help were evaluated.

Because both programs were unaffiliated with a health care treatment program, hospital, or state nursing board, the nurse seeking help was especially able to feel safe in the assessment interview. The approach of both programs with regard to confidentiality was thoroughly described at the intake interview, and program services were explained.

Information gathered included an in-depth drug and alcohol history, including inquiry into physiological withdrawal symptoms, method of obtaining drugs, presence of blackouts, multiple drug use and patterns of use (i.e., binge or daily). A detailed family history was also taken; when applicable, evaluation was made of issues related to the nurse's being an adult child of an alcoholic. Employment history was explored to assess the nurse's professional sense of competence and identification as well as the extent of any "hospital hopping," and negative consequences of drug use, such as terminations, disciplinary probations, and/or on-site arrests. The interviewer's assessment of denial and minimization of negative consequences was a part of the evaluation of the nurse's motivation for recovery and determination of the phase of chemical dependence.

Further, the initial interview focused on the nurse's previous attempts to stop alcohol or drug use by self-help, psychotherapy, or other treatment methods. This information was sought to evaluate the nurse's knowledge about chemical dependency. Many nurses seen by BATFIN and DISCOVERY had been treated by psychiatrists and/or family physicians for drug and alcohol dependency, yet continued to be addicted. Helping professionals who lack expertise in the treatment of the chemically dependent nurse often act as enablers for the addicted nurse by minimizing or denying the gravity of the nurse's drug problem.

Treatment Concerns

The need for treatment programs sensitive to the needs of addicted nurses has become increasingly evident over the last few years. The problem of chemical dependency has received little attention from the health care community, and the chemical dependency treatment community has not understood the special needs of the nurse-patient in the treatment setting. These factors have made it difficult for the chemically dependent nurse to seek appropriate treatment and support without fear of punitive consequences. Some treatment programs have counseled nurses out of the profession, suggesting they never return. Others have attempted to stop the nurse-patient from leaving treatment before planned discharge by threatening to file a report with the respective state nursing board. Still others have taken the opposite approach, encouraging nurses to return to their previous work area immediately, with access to drugs and without supervision.

Many chemical dependency treatment facilities believe that they adequately address the needs of nurses through their women's program, and do not recognize that nurses have further special needs. Specifically, a treatment program must (1) encourage the nurse to be a patient, not a helper to the other patients; (2) provide individual psychotherapy at least twice each week during in-patient treatment and once a week during out-patient treatment for a minimum of one year; (3) refer the nurse to a nurses' support group that meets at least once each week both during in-patient and out-patient treatment; (4) provide the services of a nurse consultant with expertise in the area to arrange an employment reentry contract; and (5) develop a coordinated treatment plan utilizing the psychotherapist and nurse's support group leader. Confidentiality must be maintained here; only with the nurse-patient's consent may the nurse consultant, psychotherapist, and treatment team collaborate. All other disclosures of treatment information are forbidden according to federal and state laws. The other aspects of treatment programs, such as involvement in 12-step meetings, such as Alcoholics Anonymous and Narcotics Anonymous, group sessions, family sessions, and educational lectures, as well as detoxification when necessary, are clearly aspects of treatment which are needed by the nurse addict as well.

Finally, in assessing a treatment program, it is important to look at nursing's role in the treatment team; the program nurse can provide a valuable role model for the nurse-patient, in such areas as developing relationships and coping with stress. Is the program nurse an integral part of the treatment team or merely a "baby sitter" whose input into treatment is neither valued nor sought? In addition, it is important to look at the policies and procedures of the hospital and/or treatment unit itself; how is the chemically dependent nurse there intervened with, if at all?

In addition to nurse support groups, nurse clients in the DISCOVERY program have received consultation and assistance in developing reentry contracts with their employer, psychotherapy both during in-patient treatment and on an out-patient basis, and DISCOVERY involvement in team planning during in-patient treatment. Recovering nurses visit new nurse-patients while they are in the hospital, and the nurse-patients attend weekly support group meetings at DISCOVERY during their in-patient stay. Thus, a strong support system is developed while the nurse-patient is in the hospital, which can be used after discharge.

This type of coordinated treatment approach has been the model offered by DISCOVERY, collaborating with several treatment facilities in Southern California. Currently, DISCOVERY is conducting a follow-up study of participants in its program in order to evaluate and test its program effectiveness.

Guidance Regarding Return-to-Work Issues

Members of BATFIN and DISCOVERY serve as educators and consultants to the nurse management community, to employee assistance programs, and to hospital administrators. Therefore, both program staffs know what employers expect of nurses who wish to return to the workplace after initial treatment of their chemical dependency. With their knowledge of the addictive process and the issues of recovery, BATFIN and DISCOVERY are able to design effective return-to-work contracts. These contracts protect the privacy of the nurse while providing the hospital with a reasonable tool to monitor the nurse and preserve the integrity of the health care provided. The staff of both programs are actively involved in the development of and ongoing consultation regarding the use of such contracts.

The reentry contract is between the recovering nurse and the employer. Its proposes are to provide: (1) a mechanism for monitoring job performance effectively, (2) a means to assist in identifying relapse as early as possible, (3) protection from unsubstantiated suspicion of the nurse, and (4) patient protection. BATFIN and DISCOVERY staff found that the most useful and effective contract provisions include the following:

1. attendance at recovering nurse support group meetings at least once a week;
2. twelve-step (Alcoholics Anonymous and/or Narcotics Anonymous) meetings at least four times a week;
3. completion of after-care program of the in-patient treatment program, where applicable;
4. individual psychotherapy weekly (strongly recommended);
5. random urine testing;
6. regular meetings with a work-site monitor, usually a supervisor, to discuss concerns and issues as they arise;
7. no access to narcotics, initially;
8. consultation between monitor and nurse consultant on an "as needed" basis.

We recommend that the reentry contract continue for two years, with renegotiation after one year. The staff of both programs found that one of the most important aspects of successful contract completion was preentry sessions with coworkers of the returning nurse. The sessions were conducted in order to discuss addiction in general, to provide advice on how to best support the recovering nurse, and to dispel myths and fears about the newly drug-free nurse. Coworkers are often distressed about the possibility of relapse and fearful of trusting the nurse they observed during the active phase of the disease. While specific personal issues of the returning nurse are not discussed, coworkers are encouraged to express their shock, anger, and/or resentment toward the nurse prior to the return of the nurse. Further, they are encouraged to consider their own enabling behavior. The preentry meeting or meetings provide an excellent opportunity to express feelings and prevent problems once the nurse returns to the workplace.

Nurses' Support Groups

The nurse's support group provides support, caring, and a safe place for the recovering nurse to explore issues concerning nursing, hospitals, drugs, family, life, and recovery. Many times it is the place where the nurse can be the most honest and can feel the least judged. The support also provides an opportunity for the recovering nurse to learn to socialize in a healthy way, to experiment with new ways of establishing fulfilling relationships, and to practice the expression of feelings.

The support group also provides a vehicle for education about addiction. Because nurses are health professionals, they expect and are expected by others to possess knowledge about drugs, knowledge which many feel should protect them from addiction. This dangerous myth is dispelled in group meetings as nurses share their experiences with each other. Education is also provided about relapse, an important aspect of addictive disease; prevention of relapse by increased awareness of one's own emotional traps is a frequent focus. Importantly, this group is a support group, not a therapy group, the leader's role is facilitator of group process and source of information about addiction, resources, and recovery.

Support groups generally meet once each week; DISCOVERY has conducted meetings several times weekly to accommodate differing shift schedules. We strongly recommend that support groups meet away from hospital settings, including locations identified with chemical dependency treatment. Anonymity is paramount, and, in states with mandatory reporting laws, a nurse's fear of discovery may be well justified. Support groups should be facilitated by a nurse; if the facilitator is not a recovering nurse then the group should also be co-facilitated by a recovering person with at least five years' recovery from chemical dependency in the 12-step tradition.

Members of the support group range in recovery time from a few days to several years. Those with longer recovery provide positive role models and hope for those who are new. Almost every nurse comes into treatment convinced no other nurse ever diverted a drug from the clinical setting or drank a fifth of whiskey a day. They also believe they are bad people who deserve to be punished; that is, they too believe their addiction is a moral failing rather than an illness. The nurses are amazed to discover a group of other nurses who have experienced what they have and who understand their feelings. The nurse who has successfully returned to work instills more hope in the newly recovering nurse than perhaps any other source of support.

Legal Issues

In the United States, most disciplinary action taken against nursing licenses is for drug related offenses. In addition to this administrative action, a nurse may also be subjected to criminal sanctions. The sanctions imposed on a nurse depend on whether (1) the nurse's addiction (or use) may be shown to affect job performance negatively, (2) the addicted nurse is diverting drugs from the hospital setting (most frequently the case), (3) the addicted nurse is diverting drugs so that patients are deprived of their prescribed dosage (rarely the case), (4) the state in which the nurse practices has a law requiring mandatory reporting to the state's nursing board or licensing agency, (5) the hospital calls in criminal or nursing board or consumer board investigators when its employee nurse is "caught," and (6) the state nursing board has a drug rehabilitation alternative to discipline (currently in place or being developed in at least five states).

The nurse may be charged with violations of state penal codes, health and safety codes, and/or business and professional codes, either felony or misdemeanor charges or both may be filed by the prosecutor. If found guilty, the nurse may be subject to time in jail, informal or formal probation, fines and/or community service. Sanctions imposed depend on the jurisdiction, the specific codes identified (some for instance have mandatory jail time), and the attitude of the judge toward a nurse defendant.

Administratively, state nursing boards, with authority granted by their state legislatures, may sanction a nurse's license through reprimand, license probation, or license suspension and/or revocation. Administrative sanctions generally are imposed after a finding that the nurse has demonstrated "unprofessional conduct," which is statutorily defined. This definition may include, as it does in California, a criminal conviction of an act substantially related to the practice of nursing. Thus, license discipline may result based on the criminal conviction alone, without an independent administrative finding of unprofessional conduct. The reader is referred to relevant state laws governing nursing practice as well as to codes previously mentioned that apply to nurses as well as to the lay public.

A community-based program for chemically dependent nurses must develop a legal network of attorneys familiar with the criminal and administrative sanctions applicable to these nurses. Attorneys interested in providing legal services to nurses are often available; some will also represent nurses on a sliding scale basis. BATFIN and DISCOVERY have developed such a network of attorneys who are knowledgeable about and sensitive to the issues of the recovering nurse. Special issues of the addicted health professional must be communicated to judges in order that treatment replace (or at least accompany) punishment. In addition, some criminal prosecutors are not familiar with the administrative sanctions to which the nurse is also subject; the knowledgeable defense attorney can educate here as well.

Education and Consultation

The need for education of the local health care community, the chemical dependency treatment community, and the nursing professional cannot be overstated. In response to this need, BATFIN and

DISCOVERY provide educational presentations and workshops as well as in-service education in a variety of health care settings. Lectures and panel discussions have been presented to hospital staffs, managers, administrators, employee assistance personnel, and nursing schools. Day-long workshops on the issues of the chemically dependent nurse have included treatment considerations, as well as legal information by attorneys. Topics include the disease of addiction, the scope of the problem, identification of the chemically dependent nurse, intervention techniques, and return-to-work strategies. Also included is a talk by a recovering nurse telling his/her story, which emphasizes that nurses do recover and go on to become even greater assets to their profession.

In-service education of chemical dependency treatment staff includes an overview of the problem, basic information about the nature of nursing and the nursing population, the special needs of nurse-patients, and information on how to collaborate with the community-based program staff. Attendance at treatment team meetings, as previously described, affords an excellent opportunity to educate.

Consultation by both programs has included immediate and concrete assistance to nurse managers who will call with concerns about nursing staff. In addition, consultation has been provided to staff nurses who seek help with a colleague, family members who are worried about a nurse-relative, and chemical dependency treatment staff who seek guidance about a nurse-patient who has entered their program. Ongoing consultation has been provided to nursing staffs to develop reentry contracts. Also dealt with are concerns about perceived changes in the recovering nurse's behavior and frequently expressed fears about the nurse's possible relapse.

Funding

BATFIN and DISCOVERY represent two models for operating a community-based program for chemically dependent nurses. BATFIN was a time-limited grant project, funded by a grant from the California Nurses Association (CNA). Located in the Haight Ashbury Training and Education Project in San Francisco, BATFIN was able to obtain office space, a group meeting room, and pay for staff time for two part-time employees and conduct community education and consultation. These funds from CNA also supported research and professional writing by the BATFIN staff, Marty Jessup and Millicent Buxton.

DISCOVERY has been a self-supporting program that has offered nurses support groups, psychotherapy, assessments, referral information, consultation, and education. Service have been provided on either a sliding scale basis or free of charge depending on the nurse's or institution's ability to pay. Telephone consultation to nurses, nurse managers, hospital personnel, and the public have been provided as a community service. Because of the founders' desire to make services available to every nurse seeking help, DISCOVERY's growth has been limited by financial constraints. Both the BATFIN and DISCOVERY models have the advantage of providing services free of constraints or affiliations (such as to any particular hospital or company); disadvantages include the time limits on the BATFIN grant and the financial constraints on DISCOVERY's growth.

Other models for intervention with the chemically dependent nurse exist, including peer assistance provided by many state nursing associations, primarily staffed by nurse volunteers. These programs often provide a hot-line as well as resource/referral information. Other funding models might include nurse consultation contracts with local hospitals/hospital councils to provide needed intervention services for members' nursing employees and nurse-administered out-patient programs for the chemically dependent nurse.

It is essential that these programs, once shown to be economical and highly effective at preventing relapse, be covered by insurance companies as part of an employee benefits health program. Nationally based networking to provide interstate information about services provided, including funding bases, is critical at this time. The entrepreneurial spirit can further the work of community-based organizations and agencies so that more chemically dependent nurses can be reached.

Future Research

The BATFIN and DISCOVERY programs enabled us to study the chemically dependent nurse and learn a great deal about the origins and scope of the problem, as well as the most effective means of intervention and treatment. However, many questions remain that future research must answer. For example, are there measurable predictors for the development of addiction in a nurse? If so, are they related to a positive family history of addictive disease? Another question concerns what role stress plays in the development of addiction in nurses. Further, the patterns of drug use that most nurses select should be studied. We have begun to see potential risk factors for nurses who work in critical care, who work at night, who are from addictive families, who have ready access to opiates; these factors and others must be further researched so that recommendations about prevention and intervention may be made on a solid basis of information.

Research into the stressors that nurses face is of great importance also; perhaps nursing school curricula should address issues such as grieving the death of a patient, for example. Research into the chemical dependency problem could thus have positive ramifications for the profession as a whole, not only the chemically dependent colleague. Finally, it is critical to increase our understanding and knowledge of the factors that lead a nurse to seek help; even more effective intervention and treatment programs could thus be designed.

Conclusion

The authors believe that a community-based model is unique in assisting the chemically dependent nurse. A supportive environment that provides education, referrals, and ongoing consultation is the most significant factor in determining the success of a community-based program. The profession of nursing and individual nurses must not only accept the fact that chemical dependency exists in the profession, but must work to change attitudes from moralistic denouncement to empathetic intervention. In addition, the profession must support nurse entrepreneurs who set up programs to assist the chemically dependent nurse. The autonomy of a community-based program, particularly one run or co-run by a nurse, encourages activism in calling attention to the problem in nursing schools and the profession at large.

The disadvantages of this type of program are mainly financial. Nurse entrepreneurs who initiate self-supporting nurse help programs need support from their colleagues to proceed with this type of program. We must further our sharing of experience and knowledge with other programs across the country and help to develop new programs. The authors believe we have an obligation to confront our colleagues and to challenge those beliefs and opinions that allow our addicted colleagues to remain untreated. Further, we must help hospitals develop environments in which nurses in trouble can safely ask for help; we must help them develop effective and humane policies that facilitate the nurse's entry into treatment when appropriate. Finally, we all must lobby in every state for the establishment of programs providing a therapeutic alternative to administrative sanctions. The environment is perhaps the most significant factor in determining the success of the community-based program model. The profession of nursing and nurses individually need to accept the fact that there is a problem of chemical dependency in the profession and support benevolent nurse entrepreneurs who set up programs to assist the nurse who still suffers. Community-based organizations, usually free of "political" or bureaucratic constraints placed on programs affiliated with a treatment program or a professional organization, may be activist in calling for increased attention to the problem in schools of nursing and in the profession at large, and urge treatment programs to become well-versed in the issues involved in treating a nurse for addictive disease. This level of autonomy is one extremely satisfying component of the community-based program for the impaired nurse.

Financing this type of program can be a problem; however, income may be generated by speaking and consultation fees and, to a lesser degree, by group fees and therapy fees. Foundation support may also be sought, particularly if the applicant has a good database regarding drug and alcohol problems among nurses. All fees must be on a sliding scale in order to make the program available to the greatest number of nurses in need of it.

We must start sharing our experience and knowledge with other impaired nurse programs across the country and help other nurses develop new programs. We feel we have an obligation to confront our colleagues and challenge the beliefs and opinions that allow our fellow nurses to remain hidden and sick. We must help hospitals develop an environment in which the impaired nurse may get well. We must work with hospitals to create and publicize policies that clearly state the philosophy of the hospital and what procedures will be followed for the nurse whose job performance is impaired by drugs or alcohol. Finally, as a part of our intervention, we must begin to lobby for programs that provide a therapeutic alternative to license revocation and criminal discipline in our states.

References

Board of Registered Nursing, State of California, personal communication, 1981.

Buxton, M., Jessup, M., & Landry, M. (1985). Treatment of the chemically dependent health professional. In H. B. Milkman (Ed.), *The Addictions: Multi-disciplinary Perspectives and Treatment* (pp. 131–143). Lexington, MA: Lexington Books, D. C. Heath.

Buxton, M. & Jessup, M. (1983). *A Study of 25 Nurses in Treatment.* Unpublished survey in the San Francisco Support Group for Chemically Dependent Nurses of the Bay Area Taskforce for Impaired Nurses (BATFIN).

Hardy, M. (1983). *Nurses Who Divert Drugs: An Independent Study.* Unpublished manuscript.

Sullivan, J. (1986). *Nurses In DISCOVERY.* Unpublished manuscript.

4

Florida's Alternative to Disciplinary Action

Jean T. Penny, Anne M. Catanzarite, and Judie K. Ritter

In recent years, chemical dependency has emerged as a major societal problem among people from all walks of life. Recognition of the disease as a significant issue among practitioners in the health care professions has come about largely as a result of the potentially disastrous consequences of impaired practice.

In this chapter chemical dependency is defined as "the use, misuse, abuse of and/or addiction to, any mood altering substance(s), with resulting negative consequences." This is a comprehensive definition that encompasses all stages in the progression of the disease.

There have been myriad approaches to dealing with the problem of chemically dependent nurses. Regulatory agencies such as boards of nursing have been relatively slow to respond for a variety of reasons. The main purpose of any board of nursing is to protect the public from unsafe nursing practice. Inability to practice with reasonable skill and safety due to use of alcohol or drugs is a violation of the Nurse Practice Act in most areas of the country.

This chapter describes the Intervention Project for Nurses (IPN), which represents one state board of nursing's response to the problem. The IPN is a program for chemically dependent nurses designed as an alternative to official disciplinary action by Florida's Board of Nursing.

Disciplinary Process

Historically, the only avenue available to nursing boards to ensure patient safety has been the disciplinary process. Disciplinary penalties are primarily punitive in nature and unfortunately do not address the fact that chemical dependency is a treatable disease (Barr & Learner, 1984; Bissel, Bissel & Haberman, 1984; Finley, 1982).

Specific steps in the disciplinary process employed by a given regulatory agency may vary somewhat from state to state. However, there are certain common elements. First, a complaint alleging violation of the Nurse Practice Act is filed with the state agency responsible for regulating nursing practice. Next, an investigation is conducted. A thorough review to determine the legal sufficiency of the complaint follows the investigation.

At this point, some states (such as Florida) require an additional review before a probable cause panel. The probable cause panel, composed of nurses as well as attorneys, studies all collected data relevant to the case and ascertains if there is probable cause to believe that a violation of the Nurse Practice Act has occurred. Upon a finding of probable cause, an official administrative complaint is processed and the nurse is notified of impending prosecution.

After notification, the nurse is afforded an opportunity to be heard: either at a formal hearing before an administrative hearing officer (if the nurse disputes the allegation) or at an informal hearing before the board of nursing (if the nurse does not dispute the allegations). Formal hearings are similar to regular trials except there is no jury. The hearing officer, like a judge, examines the evidence and then makes a recommendation to the board of nursing concerning the disposition of the case. The board has the option to accept, reject, or modify the recommended order based upon board members' evaluation of the entire record.

Informal hearings are conducted by boards of nursing during regularly scheduled board meetings. The nurse may testify, provide witnesses, and be represented by an attorney at both formal and informal hearings. At an informal hearing, board members determine what, if any, penalty should be imposed. Penalties may consist of a fine, a reprimand, probation, suspension, or revocation of the license. Some states have enacted "sunshine legislation" which requires that all board meetings, including disciplinary hearings, shall be open to the public.

Disciplinary proceedings are costly in terms of time, dollars, and lives. The lack of available alternative measures to ensure safe practice can lead to a double bind situation. Mandatory reporting of nurses suspected of chemical dependency results in expensive investigations, disciplinary procedures, and eventual suspension or revocation of the license rather than treatment of the disease. On the other hand, failure to report such nurses often leads to a cyclic problem of termination from one facility; subsequent employment at another; and continued jeopardy for the patient, the employing agency, and the still untreated nurse (Kelly, 1985; Penny, 1986).

Case Study #1

Joyce Taylor (fictitious name), a 23-year-old R.N., was reported to the Department of Professional Regulation by her employer in April, 1975. She had been terminated from employment with a community hospital in Florida for medication errors, incorrectly transcribing doctors' orders, and failing to chart properly. She subsequently was terminated in October, 1975 from a children's hospital for medication errors, including some that involved controlled drugs.

On January 16, 1976 an administrative complaint was issued and on April 6, 1976, Ms. Taylor was placed on probation for two years. The probation was completed on April 18, 1978.

On September 4, 1980, at a university hospital in the same area, Ms Taylor was reported to the Department of Professional Regulation, Board of Nursing for diverting Demerol® for her own use; administering a medication, Prometazine (Phenergan)®, to patients without a doctor's authorization or knowledge; and charting Demerol® as being administered to patients when in fact they were administered something other than Demerol® by Ms. Taylor.

By order of the Board of Nursing, on April 26, 1981, Ms. Taylor accepted a stipulation which included suspension of her R.N. license for one year, retroactive to September 5, 1980. Prior to application for reinstatement, she was required to undergo psychiatric counseling, complete courses in charting and legal aspects, and prove her competency to practice.

Ms. Taylor's license was reinstated and she was placed on probation for two years on February 5, 1982. She had provided the Board with documentation of psychiatric treatment.

A year later, on May 3, 1983, Ms. Taylor again was investigated for and admitted to diverting injectable Demerol for her own use from a nursing home where she was employed at the time. The Director of Nursing at the nursing home related that Ms. Taylor had been promoted to R.N. Supervisor on the 3–11 shift on April 12, 1983. The Director further stated that Ms. Taylor was an exceptional nurse, was competent, dependable, and punctual. She was the first R.N. at the nursing home center to become Employee of the Month. Knowledge of the drug diversion surfaced when another employee reported that Ms. Taylor was "not herself."

Ms. Taylor was terminated from employment at the nursing home on May 4, 1983. She subsequently was admitted to a psychiatric unit for treatment of depression.

On August 24, 1983, the Florida Board of Nursing accepted a voluntary relinquishment of license from Ms. Taylor. Before her license could be reinstated, she was required to prove her ability to practice nursing safely.

She continued with psychiatric treatment and afterwards began participating in a nurse support group. At a January, 1986 nurse support group meeting, the Director of the Intervention Project for Nurses spoke to the members. In conversation with Ms. Taylor, it was revealed that she had obtained psychiatric treatment for depression on a number of occasions, but had never received any treatment for chemical dependency. She was finally directed to an appropriate treatment program in 1986.

This actual case study is provided as an illustration of the way chemically dependent nurses were usually dealt with before the Intervention Project for Nurses was initiated.

The Advent of Alternative Programs in Regulatory Agencies

In the early 1980s it became apparent that a reevaluation of the process of disciplinary action in cases involving the chemically dependent nurse was needed. Nationally, most areas of the country were witnessing an increased incidence of nurses reported to boards of nursing for impaired practice. In Florida, joint efforts by concerned individuals, professional associations, and treatment providers laid the ground work for statutory reform.

In 1983 the Florida legislature pursuant to Chapter 464.0185 of the Florida Statutes, established authority for the Board of Nursing to develop what has become known as the IPN (Intervention Project for Nurses). The focus of Florida's IPN is on providing an alternative to disciplinary action for registered nurses and licensed practical nurses whose ability to practice is impaired by drug or alcohol abuse or a debilitating mental condition (Florida Board of Nursing, 1985). The purpose of the project is to allow nurses with no prior record of disciplinary action to enter an approved treatment facility and to be protected from disciplinary action as long as they continue to make satisfactory progress toward recovery. IPN participants can return to work after initial treatment is completed and during the two year follow-up period of monitored aftercare.

Florida has chosen to describe the IPN as an alternative program rather than a "diversion program." Diversion program is the terminology used by many authors to refer to similar programs that are also designed to divert chemically dependent nurses away from the disciplinary process and into proper treatment. However, because the word "divert" is so commonly associated with the act of illegally diverting drugs from patients, Florida prefers to identify its IPN as an alternative program.

The general philosophy of alternative (and diversion) programs maintains that chemical dependency is a disease that affects safe nursing practice. The course of the disease is most effectively altered by the appropriate treatment and continuing care. With proper treatment and monitored recovery, nurses are able to return to nursing practice without compromising patient safety or sacrificing their nursing careers.

Three other states have taken steps to develop programs that provide an alternative to traditional disciplinary action against chemically dependent nurses: California, Texas, and New York. Each of these programs differs slightly from Florida's Intervention Project for Nurses.

The California Diversion Program is operated by a Diversion Program Manager employed by the California Board of Registered Nursing. The manager acts as a liaison between the nursing board and a separate agency that is under contract to provide assessment, evaluation, referral, and monitoring services for nurses in the program. Participation is open to registered nurses and practical nurses.

The Texas Peer Assistance Program for Impaired Nurses (TPAPIN) was developed through the combined efforts of a number of voluntary nursing organizations. TPAPIN is authorized by state statute but is housed within the Texas Nurses Association, rather than an official regulatory agency. A group of trained nurse "interveners" assists in the referral of nurses to TPAPIN. Services are available for both registered nurses and licensed vocational nurses.

In New York's Committee For Professional Services, participating nurses are required to voluntarily relinquish their nursing licenses. This constitutes a form of disciplinary action and is reflected in the nurse's permanent record. Requirements for treatment and recovery are similar to the IPN. Because participation in New York's program does not actually prevent disciplinary action, it differs in this respect from a true alternative (or diversion) program.

The unique characteristic of Florida's IPN is the fact that, as mandated by law it is established within the framework of the state's official regulatory body (the Department of Professional Regulation). This feature enables the IPN to prevent or interrupt disciplinary action against a nurse's license. Only alternative programs that are established by legislation have this capacity.

History of the IPN

The IPN officially got underway in 1984 when the Department of Professional Regulation contracted with an RN to serve as the IPN Consultant. Initially the consultant focused her efforts upon helping with the development of a workable legal foundation for the program. The statutory authority and rules for the IPN are located in Chapter 464.0185, Florida Statutes and Rules Chapter 210-18.01 through 18.03, Florida Administrative Code. With the legal base in place, policies and procedures to administer the IPN could be established. These included criteria for admitting nurses to the program; monitoring compliance; approving treatment facilities; educating nurses, employers, and the public regarding the role of the IPN in managing chemical dependency (including constructive intervention strategies for employers to use when confronting a nurse with evidence of impaired practice); compiling statistical data for use in periodic reports and research projects; and handling a host of related activities that impinged upon the program. Response to the IPN was outstanding. The vast majority of nurses enrolled in the program were referred by employers.

IPN Policies and Procedures

Admission criteria for the IPN include agreement to undergo appropriate treatment at an approved treatment facility, compliance with all IPN requirements, and no prior history of disciplinary action in Florida or any other jurisdiction. A signed agreement between the nurse and the IPN specifies the following terms for voluntary participation:

1. A minimum of two years of participation.
2. Random urine screens (which may be at the nurse's expense).
3. Progress reports from the nurse every two months.
4. Progress reports by the treating professional every two months.
5. Narrative reports from the treating professional upon discharge from initial treatment, including the treatment plan.
6. Abstinence from all mood altering, controlled, or addictive substances.
7. Adherence to the Nurse Practice Act.
8. Mandatory attendance at Alcoholics Anonymous or Narcotics Anonymous meetings. Attendance at a Nurse Support Group is strongly recommended, depending upon availability of an appropriate group.

Strict confidentiality is maintained unless it should become necessary to discuss the nurse's enrollment in the program with the nurse's current or future employers. For this reason, a waiver of confidentiality is signed by all IPN nurses. Medical release forms, to provide access to medical records of all treating professionals, are also executed. Information coming directly to the IPN is not released to the Department of Professional Regulation unless the nurse fails to make satisfactory progress in the program.

When the nurse's practice is impaired due to chemical dependency, the treatment plan should be appropriate to the length and severity of the illness. A structured initial in-patient treatment period usually is recommended unless there are extraordinary extenuating circumstances. If the impairment is due to a debilitating mental condition, the treatment plan must meet the need for rehabilitation or monitoring of the condition.

Usually, when a nursing administrator suspects a nurse of chemical dependency, documentation is obtained and an intervention is planned. The nurse employer is referred to appropriate resources in the community to assist with the intervention, if help is needed. Such resources might include employee assistance programs, treatment center professionals or designated peer assistance groups. With a successful intervention, the nurse agrees to evaluation and treatment (Fulton, 1981; Jefferson & Ensor, 1982). Nurses accepted into the IPN may return to nursing practice after completion of the initial phase of treatment if their evaluations reflect stability in early recovery.

Upon reentering the workforce, IPN nurses are instructed to avoid high-stress specialty areas with easy access to drugs as well as certain shifts that might interfere with continuing care requirements (Burton & Jessup, 1982). They are required to refrain from administering controlled substances and from accepting responsibility for the keys to locked drug storage areas. Generally, employment as a nurse in a chemical dependency treatment facility is not permitted during the course of IPN participation.

The immediate supervisor must be informed of the nurse's involvement in the IPN and will be responsible for submitting periodic reports to the program concerning the nurse's progress. The employing agency may also specify additional requirements beyond those required by the IPN.

Case Study #2

The following case study exemplifies the typical approach now taken with nurses who exhibit problems with chemical dependency.

Terry Smith (fictitious name), a 31-year-old R.N., was referred to the Intervention Project for Nurses by the Director of Nursing at a major hospital in southern Florida in March, 1986. The employer expressed concern that Ms. Smith's nursing practice possibly had been affected by the use of drugs. The Director of Nurses reported that during her two year employment, Ms. Smith was a "casual" employee who floated to different units in the hospital and possessed excellent nursing skills. She also was currently working on a graduate degree in Hospital Administration.

Documentation related to practice issues included behavioral changes and a pattern of discrepancies in the charting of narcotics. This pattern was observed on all units to which she floated. Also noted were mood swings, flushed appearance, constricted pupils, and frequent absences from the unit on a number of occasions.

With the specific data, an intervention was carried out by the Director of Nurses and Ms. Smith agreed to treatment and participation in the Intervention Project for Nurses. She completed the initial (28 day) phase of treatment, and on recommendation of the treatment staff continued in extended residential treatment for six weeks.

After completion of the residential program, Ms. Smith began the continuing care (aftercare) program at the treatment center and accepted the restriction of remaining out of nursing practice for three months.

Ms. Smith was permitted to return to nursing after the three-month period. She was evaluated as stable in recovery and committed to her ongoing recovery program. She returned to her employer (who had referred her) and resumed working in the medical/surgical area. Her practice was restricted only with regard to controlled drugs: she was not able to administer controlled drugs or assume responsibility for the narcotic cabinet keys.

Terry Smith has continued to progress in her recovery. She established a relationship with the Intervention Project for Nurses when her employer referred her and continues to adhere to the requirements of the project. Reports have been received every two months to monitor her progress and continued safe practice.

During her second year of recovery, Ms. Smith resumed graduate work towards her Masters in Nursing. Her licensure record at the Board of Nursing reveals no evidence of disciplinary action.

Potential Pitfalls and Ongoing Concerns

Inasmuch as there was no role model or prototype for the IPN to follow, project development has necessarily been evolutionary in nature. Based on the experience of the IPN's first year of operation, the need for certain changes in focus became apparent. For example, a decision was made to shift the function of actually monitoring participants' progress to the treatment professionals responsible for their care. Conceptually, it is more appropriate for treatment personnel than IPN staff to monitor progress because of the treatment professionals' clinical expertise and their close contact with clients. Their around the clock availability can become a critical factor in the event of an emergency.

It was important to recognize, too, the potential for conflict if IPN personnel were perceived by project participants or by treatment professionals as providing any form of therapy or "hands on" care. Staff members serve in an advisory capacity only. As facilitators, they concentrate their efforts on coordinating the educational and administrative aspects of the project in an effort to ensure the best possible use of available resources.

For example, IPN staff activities include evaluation and approval of treatment facilities according to IPN standards. Consultation is provided for employers and others regarding proper interface with the program. Referrals are made to resources in local communities. Educational seminars and workshops are provided upon request throughout the state and across the nation. Ongoing efforts center on problem solving; data collection and analysis; information sharing; and refining the components of the intervention, treatment; and aftercare processes.

The IPN maintains a close and interdependent working relationship with the Florida Board of Nursing and the Department of Professional Regulation relative to reporting, investigations, probable cause reviews, disciplinary hearings, or other actions involving IPN nurses. This is vital to the mission of the IPN as it is the official alignment with the department that gives the program the authority to affect licensure status.

During the second year of operation, dialogue ensued regarding the need for a name change. Originally, the IPN was called the Impaired Nurse Program (INP). It was decided that a name change was in order because of the negative connotation associated with labeling participating nurses "impaired." The nurse's practice may be impaired due to the effects of chemical dependency, but with successful treatment, the individual can return to normal functioning. Further, on a philosophical level recovering nurses objected to continued identification with a project designated for "impaired nurses."

The name "Intervention Project for Nurses" was selected because of the more positive message it conveys. Also, it can be abbreviated with the same three initials as the INP (except in a different order) which served to reduce confusion during the period of transition.

Procedures to deal with nurses who suffer relapses were not in place at the beginning of the program. This was a potentially serious weakness since relapses, like denial, are characteristic of the disease of chemical dependency. Now, as a matter of course, the relapsing nurse immediately takes a leave of absence from practice and returns to the treatment facility for a total reevaluation. Recommendations for further treatment are made at that time. Then, the nurse's file is reviewed by the board's probable cause panel and a determination is made whether or not the nurse can continue in the IPN without disciplinary action. Factors considered in making this determination include the length and severity of the relapse, treatment professionals' recommendations, prior history of relapses, and so forth. At present, this is a trial procedure under evaluation. It is an ongoing challenge to find the most effective means to deal therapeutically with the recovering nurse and yet, at the same time, assure that the safety of health care consumers is not compromised.

It was initially thought that limiting IPN eligibility to nurses with no prior history of disciplinary action would serve to increase the likelihood of meeting program objectives. This stance did not take into consideration, however, the increase in reporting of chemically dependent nurses that would occur as a result of the availability of a viable alternative to disciplinary action. Nor did it consider the increased number of requests for assistance from nurses who had not had the benefit of such an alternative previously.

From a humanistic perspective, it seems inconsistent to deny a nurse services provided by the project (such as referral for treatment, linkage with support groups, etc.) because of disciplinary action taken in the past. IPN staff are investigating measures to increase project services for such nurses and also to improve the availability of treatment options.

Another ongoing concern is related to funding. Currently, the IPN is funded by the legislature on a year-to-year basis. This means that there is the potential for turnovers among elected officials in state government to have an influence on the interest in and therefore the amount of support for programs similar to the IPN. The fact that the IPN has extensive grassroots support among the professional community and has received much favorable national attention as well should work in favor of continued backing from the legislature, regardless of political changes.

Statistics and Strengths

The IPN staff consists of three registered nurses, the consultant who directs the program, and two coordinators. There is one clerical support person. At the end of 3½ years of operation, there are 500 nurses enrolled in the project and 130 have completed participation.

The IPN advocates the theory that the need to preserve licensure probably plays as strong a role in motivating some chemically dependent nurses to seek treatment as the desire to recover their health (Naegle, 1985). This factor undoubtedly helps promote compliance with IPN requirements. Further, it is felt that housing the IPN under the same umbrella agency that is responsible for regulating nursing practice may result in better control over administering the program than is possible under any other circumstances. In the event of noncompliance, for example, the IPN's ability to swiftly initiate steps to prevent further clinical practice by that nurse serves as a mechanism to increase the protection of the public from unsafe practitioners.

The IPN has been described as a classic example of a "win–win" arrangement. The health care consumer wins because a potentially dangerous situation is averted when a chemically dependent nurse withdraws from practice. After appropriate treatment, the nurse wins because recovery has been affected without disciplinary action or loss of licensure (W. Furlow, 1986, personal communication).

The issue of dealing with chemically dependent nurses, from the Florida Board of Nursing's regulatory agency viewpoint, is threefold. First and foremost, there is an obligation to protect the public from unsafe practice by assuring that nurses whose judgement and capability are impaired do not endanger the lives or well-being of health care consumers. Secondly, there is a humanitarian concern to recognize and treat chemical dependency as a disease process and thereby to conserve the valuable resource that nurses represent in society. Finally, there is a need to reduce the negative impact of this pervasive problem upon the integrity of the nursing profession as a whole.

The IPN has served as a vehicle to enable the Board to address these concerns officially. This innovative program has enhanced Florida nurses' credibility by demonstrating that they are willing to accept responsibility and be held accountable for a creative solution to a difficult professional problem.

References

Barr, M., & Lerner, W. (1984). The impaired nurse: A management issue. *Nursing Economics, 2,* 196–201.

Bissell, L., & Haberman, P. (1984). *Alcoholism in the professions.* New York: Oxford University Press.

Burton, M., & Jessup, M. (1982). Nurses' support group. *Hospital Employee Health.* 24–25.

Finley, B. (1982). Secondary prevention of substance abuse in nurses. *Occupational Health Nursing, 30*(11), 14–18.

Florida Board of Nursing. (1985). *Impaired nurse program.* (Public document). Jacksonville, FL.

Fulton, K. (1981). What nursing management can do. *Supervisor Nurse, 22*(1), 18–20.

Furlow, W. (1986, April). Senior Prosecuting Attorney, Department of Professional Regulation, State of Florida. Unpublished comments to the Florida Board of Nursing.

Jefferson, L., & Ensor, B. (1982). Confronting a chemically dependent colleague. *American Journal of Nursing, 82*(4), 572–577.

Kelly, R. (1985). Rx: Swifter help for the chemically dependent nurse. *American Journal of Nursing. 85*(6), 640–642.

Naegle, M. (1985). Creative management of impaired nursing practice. *Nursing Administration Quarterly, 9*(3), 16–26.

Penny, J. (1986). Spotlight on support for impaired nurses. *American Journal of Nursing, 86*(6), 688–691.

5

Employee Assistance Programs: A Key to Early Identification and Treatment

Lorraine Hall

Health care administrators, concerned about cost containment, have become increasingly aware of the importance of effectively managing their human resources. In particular reference to nurses, the present work force is aging and there are fewer applicants to nursing schools to replace them since young people today have more vocational choices than a decade ago. UCLA's Higher Education Research Institute polls (National study, 1987, cited in *AJN News*, 1987) conducted in 1986 showed that only 5.1% of freshmen women are choosing nursing, down from 8.4% in 1983. This decline is the most substantial reported in any three-year period. In addition, in a recent study (Haack, 1987) 14% of nursing students reported that alcohol use had interfered with work and school and more than 50% scored in the high range of burnout.

The American Nurses' Association estimates that 6 to 8% of registered nurses have a substance abuse problem (American Nurses' Association, 1987). It, therefore, makes good economic and professional sense to establish methods of identifying new graduates with

The author gratefully acknowledges the assistance of Nancy MacDonald for the research in the preparation of this chapter.

alcohol and drug abuse problems as well as those experienced professionals already in the work place. Employee Assistance Programs (EAPs) are increasingly being recognized as an effective approach for the identification and treatment of employees in a variety of work settings.

As administrators of health care facilities become more aware of the success of Employee Assistance Programs in private industry and business, they have begun to examine how the EAP model might be adapted to meet the particular needs of their employees, especially their valued nursing group. EAPs are designed to help the employee identify, confront, and resolve long-term personal or family problems by providing a confidential and convenient "one stop" resource for information, problem assessment, motivation, and referral to the most effective resource in the community.

EAPs are designed to be a "safe haven," a place where on a self-referral basis, employees can discuss a problem with a professional and receive confidential assistance without management being informed. It can be viewed as an extra employee benefit—a personal consultation service available if and when the need arises.

The employee assistance program can also be used by management and labor unions as an effective tool in resolving job performance problems. Representing an average of 25% of all referrals to an EAP (Rhode Island Employee Assistance Program, 1987), the management or supervisor referral carries a much greater share of the return-on-investment (ROI) justification for an employee assistance program. An employer has the right to require change if an employee's behavior or job performance standards are not acceptable (Fulton, 1981). If a personal problem is the cause of the job performance problem, the employee may be offered the assistance of the EAP for assessment and referral to appropriate treatment. If the employee's sense of self-worth is closely linked to the job and job performance is questioned, the employee may respond well to an offer of assistance by the EAP. It is the author's experience that nurses are particularly responsive to this appeal, once it is clear that whatever efforts they have made on their own have not succeeded.

Recovery rates from chemical dependency are practically identical whether the person sought help on a self-referral basis or was referred by a concerned supervisor because of deteriorating job performance. A four-year follow-up study of 218 Textron, Inc. employees referred for alcoholism treatment revealed a recovery rate of 82% (based on abstinence and significant improvement in life-functioning). Of this total group, 157 (72%) were self-referrals and 61 (28%) were supervisor referrals; each had the same rate of recovery (82%) (MacDonald, 1985).

This chapter will briefly review the history of EAPs and particular problems of implementation with a health care workforce, as well as demonstrate how the establishment of an EAP can be an effective means of reaching the troubled or chemically dependent nurse.

History of the Employee Assistance Movement

The forerunners of today's comprehensive EAPs go back to the 1940s: in fact, the New England Telephone Company started an Alcohol Assistance Program in 1939 (Employee Assistance Programs, 1981). Major companies throughout the United States followed with efforts aimed primarily at dealing with alcoholism in the work place, still the primary problem for today's EAPs (Dubreuil & Krause, 1983). There was little knowledge of or treatment resources for alcoholism, and as such responsible employers saw these programs as a solution to the frustrating problem of what to do about the once-valued employee who seemed to be on a self-destructive course. These early occupational alcohol programs (OAPs) succeeded, and they managed to save the careers, marriages, and even the lives of many an employee.

In the 1960s and 1970s, these programs began to broaden their scope to include other long-term physical, emotional, marital, and family problems that were of concern to and affecting the performance of employees (Dubreuil & Krause, 1983). They also recognized that the problems of a family member could affect the employee's well being and performance as much as a personal problem. Thus, assistance was also offered to family members.

These programs became known as "broad brush" EAPs—comprehensive services that provided a certain degree of anonymity, in that clients were not identified as "alcoholic" or "crazy" by their use of the EAP. They also provided a "safe" way for alcoholics to seek help initially for a "marriage problem" or "stress problem." A skilled EAP counselor can assess the use or abuse of alcohol and other drugs and will uncover the role these substances play in the presenting problem.

In the 1970s in response to the needs of female workers as well as to those of middle or senior management (almost all of whom were male), major employee assistance programs began to examine not only the content of their services but the methods by which these services were presented to supervisors or employee groups (Masi, 1984; Wrich, 1980). As an example of these efforts, Textron, Inc., with a well-known employee assistance program covering 46,000 employees in 26 states, embarked on a major effort to increase utilization of the EAP by female employees. Literature and training material were revised to remove any sex bias and to emphasize assistance for problems of greater concern to female employees: stress of dual careers or single parenting, co-dependency issues of alcoholism in the household, behavioral problems of children, family violence, and financial problems.

In addition, supervisor training at the Textron facilities sensitized supervisors, especially males, to their enabling behavior toward female employees versus a more confrontive attitude toward male workers who had identical job performance problems. Elimination of the double standard and emphasis on correcting job performance problems by utilizing the EAP as a management tool or resource dramatically increased supervisor referrals of women to the program. Once referred, whether as a self-referral or as a supervisor referral, the female worker was, in most cases, assisted by a female EAP coordinator recruited as part of the total effort by Textron to respond to the needs of women in the workplace.

As a result of these efforts, women accounted for 32% of all employees seeking services from the EAP, matching exactly the percentage of female employees in their workforce at that time (MacDonald, 1981).

Today, it is estimated that over 10,000 employers in the United States have employee assistance programs (Bureau of National Affairs, 1986), but health care institutions are not well represented in this group. For instance, an American Hospital Association survey found that fewer than one-third of all hospitals provided EAP services for their workforces. In response to this dearth of EAPs, Kabb (1984) advocated funding EAPs for hospital settings not only to provide a system of responding to deteriorating job performance, but as a major effort aimed at preventing such problems. The benefits of EAPs, such as reducing absenteeism, excessive use of costly health care benefits, inappropriate workers' compensation claims, high staff turnover rates, and costly mistakes, have been widely discussed, as have the broader aims of improved morale, better employee relations and the retention of skilled, experienced professionals. Since hospitals employ 68% of nurses and nursing homes and extended care facilities employee another 8% (DHHS, 1986, p. 112), implementing EAPs in just these settings would provide systematic assistance to a majority of the practicing nurses in the United States (Blair, 1985). Unfortunately, the advocates of establishing EAPs in health care settings are not always heard.

The Health Care Institution—Barriers to Establishment of Employee Assistance Programs

Barriers to the establishment of EAPs in health care institutions are various. Some individuals or nursing departments believe that EAPs will cause them to "lose control" over their employees. Others believe they can "take care of their own" (Landesman & Bucolo, 1987) or meet the needs of all employees in the institution. Yet others' concerns are based on the financial cost to the institution for implementation of such a program (Blair, 1985) and fears of civil action against supervisors, peers, or institutions (Naegle, 1985).

Some less enlightened administrators also fear the public will perceive an employee assistance program as a coverup of some possible serious wrongdoings by the staff or as a "soft" way of dealing with troubled employees, although the contrary is true. The EAP aims to resolve problems by retaining valued, experienced professionals, rather than terminating them without a chance to address and correct their problems; however, the EAP does not preclude normal disciplinary action.

The nursing profession must adjust to today's job market, where the pool of nurses from which to draw staff is decreasing. Even without this consideration, a high turnover rate is an expensive way to run an institution. Health care facilities must find ways to stabilize their largest single workgroup — nursing personnel. There is reason to believe that the establishment of EAPs in health care institutions will give the same return on investment realized by private business and industry for many years. Sullivan (1986) describes these savings as reduction of replacement costs, selection, and orientation and training, conservatively estimated at $3,000 per employee.

Finally, hospital administrators and nurses themselves must put aside the misconception that nurses, by virtue of their education and training, are somehow better able to solve their own personal or family problems or, worse yet, that they are invulnerable to the onslaught of chemical dependency. Nurses experience the same frailties, fears, frustrations, and susceptibility to the use, abuse, or addiction to mood altering substances as other individuals. In fact, nurses are believed to be at a higher risk because they know which drugs may "work" for them during a time of stress or exhaustion, and these drugs are accessible in the workplace. In addition nurses have the pressures of critical patient care, erratic work schedules, and demanding responsibilities.

Employee Assistance Programs are an option for professional nursing organizations who are seeking a way to professionally staff and manage Peer Assistance Programs. For instance, the Colorado State Nurses' Association and Rhode Island State Nurses' Association (Hall, 1986) have formal contractual arrangements with private, nonprofit EAPs. The cost of the contracts is funded by the respective state divisions of substance abuse. Other methods of funding could include membership assessment, grants from private sector foundations, or direct contributions to the program.

Choosing an EAP for a Health Care Setting

An EAP may be advocated by an advisory committee, the personnel department, employee health clinic, a wellness committee, a risk management group, a nursing, social work, or psychiatric department, or any combination of these. Wherever the advocacy begins, it is essential that top administrative staff and union officials, if a union exists, be involved in the process of planning, choosing, promoting, and insuring the political survival of the EAP (Blair, 1985).

A decision must also be made about program design, which is most commonly either an internal model or external provider model. With the internal model, the EAP professionals are employees of the health care institution; the EAP may be run by a particular department of a hospital such as social services (Lesser & Cavaseno, 1986), psychiatry, or personnel health (O'Connor & Robinson, 1985). The advantages of an internal EAP program are accessibility, sensitivity to internal politics, and knowledge of the work environment. The internal EAP professional is quickly available for management of crisis situations. Changes in EAP policies may also be accomplished more readily. Disadvantages include employee concerns about confidentiality, a key program component. Cost is also a negative factor; the EAP professional must be paid a salary and benefits, an office must be supplied and furnished, and support services must be provided for the program. If an EAP is set up within an existing hospital department, it may be more difficult to provide an *objective* assessment for employees who are also coworkers.

The external provider model provides services on a contractual basis. The provider may be a professional EAP organization, community mental health center, a hospital, or a family service agency. Fees are negotiated according to services provided, either on a per capita or fee-for-service basis.

One advantage of an externally provided EAP is that it enables smaller health care settings without resources for an internal program to obtain EAP services. Also, an outsider provider may be viewed by employees as providing more confidentiality than an internal program. Staff members and expertise may also be more varied than with an internal program. In addition, salary and benefit costs as well as overhead costs are spread out across the many client employers served by the EAP provider, usually at 1/2 or 1/3 the cost of an internal program.

In evaluating a prospective EAP, the health care institution should look for a provider with experience in the health care setting. Newcomers to the field of EAPs may be unprepared for the complexities of dealing with the many occupational levels in the health care workforce: managerial, professional, technical, and support services workers, all of whom present vastly different case management problems.

Whichever model is considered, the EAP professionals(s) or provider must demonstrate the ability to work with licensed professionals, since they will constitute the largest work group within the institution. The EAP must be able to deal with issues of liability, fitness for duty (Wu, Martens, & Deger, 1984), back-to-work contracts following chemical dependency treatment, and special concerns of women. The EAP must also be able to train nurse managers in the recognition and documentation of job indicators that signal unresolved personal problems, with special attention to chemical dependency markers (Bissell, 1984; Cross, 1985; Cyster, 1986; Doyle, 1986; Jefferson & Ensor, 1982; Naegle, 1985).

The EAP must be sensitive to the special stigma felt by women with personal problems, and must develop techniques to encourage self-referrals to the program (Pape, 1987; Solomon, 1983). Because a significant proportion of employee problems will be alcohol or drug related, *the EAP provider, whether internal or external, must have a staff with expertise in chemical dependency.*

Once an EAP is chosen, publicized, and implemented, in-service programs on special topics, such as stress management or single parenting, keep the EAP program and staff visible.

Implementation of an EAP

First, senior hospital management and union officials, in acknowledging the value of an EAP as an employee benefit, a cost containment vehicle, and as a management tool for resolving job performance problems, must show visible support for the program by attending training events, introducing the EAP presenters at employee sessions, communicating the program to all subordinates, and mandating attendance at all presentations.

Confidentiality of the EAP must be emphasized. Simply stated (and it should be stated often), if a person seeks help on a self-referral basis, no one in hospital management, the union or anyone else, will be notified. It should also be made clear to employees that EAP records are kept separate from personnel records.

If a person is referred by management as a result of job performance issues, the employee will be asked to sign a release for information about acceptance of and compliance with the treatment plan to be given to the appropriate management or supervisory referral personnel. Absolutely no information is given out as to the nature of the problem or treatment resources that could identify the nature of the problem.

Another area of crucial importance to the success of an EAP is supervisor training. Supervisors are taught not to diagnose the problem, confront the problem with the employee or, try to fix the problem by counseling the employee or finding helping resources and referring the employee themselves. These are all well-meaning and normal responses to a peer or employee, however, they are rarely successful.

A system for evaluating the effectiveness of the EAP must be part of the service agreement with the provider. Utilization rate, analysis of utilization respective to the employee demographics, and user satisfaction surveys are common methods used. The evaluation process also serves to identify problem areas, such as maintaining visibility with professional staff who work on off-shifts or helping employees from upper and middle level management.

Reaching the Impaired Nurse Through an EAP

Nurses whose job performance is adversely affected by the misuse of drugs or alcohol are often protected by well-meaning supervisors and coworkers. This protection sometimes continues for long periods of time allowing the nurse to become increasingly dysfunctional and a threat to patient well-being and safety. Supervisors, by virtue of their training as nurses, also often enable the problem to become progressively worse by attempting to diagnose it, to intervene themselves, or to treat the problems. When supervisors "switch hats" or roles from friend, to professional, to supervisor and back again, they can unknowingly enable the troubled nurse to avoid help by manipulating the system to conceal the possible addiction.

No one intends to become an alcoholic or an addict. Every chemically dependent nurse has a different story to tell: a "pick-me-up" after an exhausting shift, an escape from an overwhelming family problem, recreational use without a thought of the consequences, a gradual dependence, or a sudden plunge into the world of addiction. The stories may vary, but the results are the same: a lonely, frightened person who more than likely will initially refuse help.

Documentation

Denial is the hallmark symptom of chemical dependency, so supervisors of nurses should not attempt to diagnose the nature of the troubled employee's problem. Kabb (1984) advises staying focused on job performance indicators: attendance, late arrivals/ early departures, requests for assignment changes, employee health/emergency room visits, on-the-job accidents/incidents, complaints by staff/patients, and comparison of written performance reviews.

Table 5.1 offers guidelines developed by the author to aid the documentation of changes (Rhode Island Employee Assistance Program, 1985).

Evaluation Guidelines

Most major health, life, or addiction problems become progressively worse if untreated and they eventually will be reflected in increasing problems on the job. When using the preceding list, a great number of items need not be checked to indicate a problem; the greater the number checked, the more probable a problem exists. Also, a chemical dependency problem will likely continue and worsen despite the promises and efforts of the troubled nurse to improve.

Intervention

After gathering sufficient objective evidence, the nursing supervisor may alert the EAP counselor that an intervention is going to be held, and that a referral will be made. The EAP counselor may choose to keep a time slot open to see the nurse for an evaluation immediately after the intervention.

The nursing supervisor and another management person then call the nurse in for a meeting and confront the troubled nurse in a con-

TABLE 5.1 Checklist For Detecting Potential Chemical Dependence in an Employee

1. Absenteeism
______a. Frequent unscheduled short-term absences
______b. Higher absenteeism rate than other employees for colds, flu, gastritis, etc.
______c. Absences after payday or days off
______d. Inconsistent or increasingly improbable excuses for absences
______e. Absences for traffic or home accident injuries

2. "On-the-job" Absenteeism
______a. Long coffee breaks
______b. Physical illness on the job (frequent trips to Employee Health Department)
______c. Excessive time for charting/record keeping
______d. "Locked door syndrome"—excessively long use of rest room

3. Difficulty in Concentration
______a. Assignment takes more time (despite skill/experience)
______b. Difficulty in assigning priorities in clinical caseload
______c. Medication errors (wrong medication, wrong dose, administration to wrong patient)
______d. Omitted, illogical, incomplete, or illegible charting
______e. Deteriorating handwriting during shift
______f. Errors in transcribing orders or taking verbal orders
______g. Overlooking signs of a patient's deteriorating condition

4. Inconsistent Work Patterns
______a. Alternate periods of high and low efficiency
______b. Becoming or has become less dependable
______c. Doing minimnal or substandard work in comparison with peers
______d. Frequent requests for help with patient assignments

5. Physical/Emotional Problems
______a. Changes in physical/emotional condition during shift
______b. Marked nervousness on the job
______c. Excessive sweating
______d. Tremors of hands
______e. Lack of attention to personal cleanliness or grooming
______f. Reports to duty despite physical or emotional contraindication

6. Decreasing Job Efficiency
______a. Omits treatments
______b. Makes bad decisions or shows poor judgment
______c. Lacks usual initiative or enthusiasm
______d. Requests change to less supervised shift

TABLE 5.1 continued

7. Poor Relationships on the Job
______a. Wide swings in mood from isolation to angry outbursts
______b. Uncooperative with coworkers
______c. Avoids contact with nurse-leader or supervisor
______d. Complaints by patients of irritability, physical roughness, or verbal abuse

8. Medication-Centered Problems
______a. Frequently around medication cart or closet
______b. Increased p.r.n. psychoactive medications or narcotics recorded for patients
______c. Increase in wastage/breakage of controlled substances
______d. Missing drugs, unaccounted doses
______e. Seeks out on-duty physicans for personal complaints of pain, backache, migraines, etc.

9. Personal Life Interferes With Job
______a. Frequent or excessively long phone calls
______b. "Visitors" on unexplained errands during work shift

cerned but firm manner. They identify the job performance issues while maintaining the self-esteem of the individual. Clearly documented facts are presented to the nurse, administrative or disciplinary action is explained, and, most importantly, an offer of assistance is made to the troubled nurse. A simplified dialogue might go as follows:

> Betty, you've been one of the best nurses on this floor and I could always depend upon you, but lately I've been observing a number of major job infractions (present facts). Due to the seriousness of these problems, I'm recommending that (appropriate disciplinary action). However, if there's an outside problem in your life that's causing these problems on the job, the hospital now has an employee assistance program that can help with those problems. I'd be willing to make a referral for you . . . the help is confidential and I will not be told the nature of the problem. However, I will be informed as to your compliance with the recommendations of the EAP. If you follow through and your performance improves, we'll hold on this action.

It is an offer that's difficult to refuse, and few do. Once the employee accepts, the supervisor notifies the EAP and an appointment is made for a confidential assessment. The employee will not have to divulge the nature of the personal problem to the supervisor or to peers. Self-esteem and morale can be enhanced by the fact that management cared enough about the nurse as a professional and a person to offer this help.

It is the responsibility of the EAP staff professional to build a trusting relationship, ask the right questions, dispel any myths or misunderstandings about chemical dependency, determine the sort of treatment or assistance needed, motivate the nurse to accept help, and make referrals to treatment professionals or programs responsive to the needs of health care professionals. An important role of the EAP counselor is the determination of appropriate treatment modalities, for example, in-patient or out-patient treatment. If in-patient treatment is required, the EAP counselor advises the nursing administrator that a medical leave of absence is required, and ideally the appropriate health care insurance pays for treatment.

It is the responsibility of the EAP to monitor the employee's progress through treatment by weekly contact with the treatment provider as well as through scheduled contact with the nurse. Progress, or lack of it, is reported back to the referring supervisor and/or responsible personnel manager, after the necessary releases of information have been signed by the nurse.

Reentry

Ideally, nursing management, the recovering nurse, and the EAP counselor collaborate on a plan of reentry into the work place by the recovering nurse. Robbins (1987) advocates the use of a Monitored Treatment Program, contained within the EAP, and a Return to Work Contract. The contract could include these core statements as well as others relevant to the particular recovering nurse's case (Robbins, 1987; Sullivan, 1986):

> I will refrain from using any mood-altering chemicals, unless such chemicals are required as part of my medical care and substantiated in writing by my primary care physician.
>
> I will agree to chemical monitoring of urine and/or blood weekly, and random testing as requested by my supervisor.

I agree to follow the aftercare treatment plan outlined and be monitored by my EAP counselor.

If I do not comply, either in attendance or documentation, I will be terminated from employment and I will be reported to the State Board of Nursing.

The contract should be signed by the nurse, the administrator, and the EAP counselor.

Although this contract may seem restrictive, in fact, it is very effective. The Texas Peer Assistance Program for Impaired Nurses studied 50 nurses who reentered the workplace with a return to work contract and found that 81% successfully complied with the terms of the agreement (Alexander, 1987).

In addition to EAP monitoring and contractual agreement, other workplace adjustments may also be made. The nurse who is recovering from addiction to drugs may be restricted from administering controlled substances usually for at least the first 6 to 12 months. When the nurse resumes administration of controlled substances, a peer monitor may be designated to supervise for a period of time. Day shift work is recommended, as supervision is most often easier to arrange. To decrease the returning nurse's stress, the nurse manager may assign the nurse to a less hectic unit but should avoid, if possible, assigning a unit that does not utilize the nurse's full capabilities (Robbins, 1987).

Summary

The EAP in the healthcare setting, in collaboration with nursing management, can ensure the most effective methods of identifying the impaired nurse, arrange for appropriate treatment, and guide the nurse's reentry into the workplace. The partnership successfully retains the recovering nurse within the profession while protecting the client and the institution.

References

Alexander, D. (1987, March). *The effectiveness of the return-to-work contract on the recovery of the impaired nurse.* Paper presented at the 5th National Impaired Nurse Symposium and Research Conference, Atlanta, GA.

American Nurses' Association. (1987, March). Impaired nursing practice (media backgrounder). *ANA News,* Kansas City: Communications Unit, Division of Marketing and Public Affairs.
Blair, B. (1985). *Hospital Employee Assistance Programs.* Chicago: American Hospital Publishing, Inc.
Bissell, L. (1984). *Alcoholism in the professions.* New York: Oxford University Press.
Bureau of National Affairs. (1986). *Alcohol and drugs in the workplace: cost, controls and controversies.* Washington, D. C.: The Bureau of National Affairs, Labor Special Projects Unit.
Cross, L. (1985). Chemical dependency in our ranks: Managing a nurse in crisis. *Nursing Management 11,* 15–16.
Cyster, R. (1986). Alcoholism. Setting limits. *Nursing Times,* May 7–13, 51–55.
Doyle, S. (1986). How managers can help. *Nursing Life,* 6(3), 42.
Dubreuil, E., & Krause, N. (1983). Employee assistance programs: Industrial and clinical perspectives. In S. W. White (ed.), *New Directions for Mental Health Services,* pp. 85–94. San Francisco: Jossey-Bass.
Employee Asistance Programs. A dollars and sense issue. (1981, November). Newport Beach, CA: Comprehensive Care Corporation.
Fulton, K. (1981). Drug abuse among nurses. What nursing management can do. *Supervisor Nurse, 1,* 18–20.
Haack, M. (1987). Alcohol use and burnout among student nurses. *Nursing & Health Care, 8*(4), 238–242.
Hall, L. (1986). Rhode Island's contract for employee assistance. *American Journal of Nursing, 86*(6), 690.
Jefferson, L. V., & Ensor, B. E. (1982). Confronting a chemically impaired colleague. *American Journal of Nursing, 82*(4), 574–577.
Kabb, G. M. (1984). Chemical dependency. Helping your staff. *The Journal of Nursing Administration, 11,* 18–23.
Landesman, T., & Bucolo, J. (1987). EAPs in health care. *EAP Digest, 1–2, 37–39.*
Lessor, J. G., and Cavaseno, V. (1986). Establishing a hospital's employee assistance program. *Health and Social Work, 11*(2), 126–132.
MacDonald, R. (1981). *Utilization Review*—Supplement to *Textron Human Resources Report.* Providence: Textron, Inc.
MacDonald, R. W. (1985). *Treatment outcome study-Northeast. Human Resources Report.* Providence: Textron, Inc.
Masi, D. A. (1984). *Designing Employee Assistance Programs.* New York: American Management Associations.
Naegle, M. (1985). Creative management of impaired nursing practice. *Nursing Administration Quarterly, 9*(2), 16–26.

National Study shows sharp drop of college freashman planning nursing careers. (1987). *American Journal of Nursing, 87*(4), 530–531.

O'Connor, P., & Robinson, R. (1985). On the scene at the Unviersity of Cincinnati Hospital. *Nursing Administration Quarterly, 9*(2), 31–68.

Pape, P. (1987, May). *Superwoman and other stereotypes.* Paper presented at the 33rd International Institute on the Prevention and Treatment of Alcoholism, Lausanne, Switzerland.

Rhode Island Employee Assistance Program. (1987, April). Quarterly report. Warrick: Robert MacDonald.

Robbins, C. (1987). A monitored treatment program for impaired health care professionals. *The Journal of Nursing Administration, 7*(2), 17–21.

Solomon, S. (1983) Women in the workplace. *Alcohol Health and Research World, 7*(3), 3–5.

Sullivan, E. (1986). Cost savings of retaining chemically dependent nurses. *Nursing Economics, 4*(4), 179–182,200.

U. S. Department of Health and Human Services. (1986, June). *The registered nurse population—findings from the national sample survey of registered nurses.* Washington, D. C.: Evalyn B. Moses.

Wrich, J. T. (1980). *The employee assistance program updated for the 1980s.* Center City, MN: Hazelden.

Wu, A. F., Martens, L. C., & Deger, P. (1984). The merits of a fitness-for-duty policy. *Hospitals, 9*(1), 78–80.

6

The Process of Recovery: Chemically Dependent Nurses

Eileen Zungolo and Carol Bowers

Consideration of Treatment Approaches for the Chemically Dependent Nurse

Having identified and effectively intervened with the impaired nurse, crucial decisions need to be made in order to provide the nurse with the maximum opportunity to achieve recovery. This chapter presents an overview of treatment services available for chemical dependency and the relative advantages and disadvantages of varying formats as they attempt to meet the needs specific to health professionals.

Since there are a number of controversial issues within the field of addiction that have profound impact on the perception of treatment and its outcome, it seems important to clarify for the reader certain beliefs of the authors.

1. We believe chemical dependency is a disease caused by multiple interacting and cumulative factors of physiological, biochemical, neurological, psychological, and social origin.
2. We believe a *minimum* behavioral goal of treatment is total abstinence from any substance that possesses mood-altering properties.

Underlying these beliefs is the concept of a *process* of recovery. Just as an individual becomes psychologically and/or physiologically dependent over time, so the chemically dependent person goes through certain phases along the path to sobriety. Since these phases have characteristic features that must be addressed in treatment, they can provide an organizing structure for this discussion.

For the purpose of this chapter the stages of recovery are labeled and defined as follows:

1. Detoxification: period of time from entry into treatment with abstinence to the cessation of physical withdrawal symptoms.
2. Initial sobriety: 7 to 10 days after detoxification.
3. Transition* phase: first month following initial sobriety.
4. Early recovery: period of time following transition until one year of abstinence.
5. On going recovery: continuous abstinence from mood-altering chemicals.

The above delineation is very arbitrary and clearly focuses only on the time dimension. Nonetheless, this approach can be functional within this context since length of abstinence, in and of itself, brings about certain changes in the client. Although these changes are highly individualistic, there are commonalities around which treatment interventions can be organized and, in fact, which may determine treatment depending on the treatment milieu.

It is fallacious to consider treatment alternatives as occurring either in an in-patient or an out-patient setting. Ideally, the chemically dependent nurse will participate in a comprehensive treatment plan that takes advantage of the full range of treatment options as necessary, from intensive acute detoxification in an in-patient environment to family counseling on an as-needed basis during ongoing recovery.

If such a plan is to be implemented successfully, the following assessments must be made as the chemically-dependent nurse approaches each phase of recovery:

*Transition is the label used by Brown (1985) to refer to the period of time initially following cessation of drinking.

1. The nurse's status, including all dimensions of the disease process—physiological, biochemical, neurological, psychological, and social.
2. Advantages and disadvantages of in-patient and out-patient treatment in relation to the nurse's total lifestyle, including threats to sobriety and factors impinging on professional rehabilitation.

The reader needs to bear in mind that out-patient care is offered across a very broad continuum. Intensive out-patient programs commonly meet on a daily basis from 3 to 5 hours, either during the day or evening. Other nonintensive formats may include daily, or two or more sessions on a weekly basis. Some nurses seek treatment by attending only one or fewer sessions a week.

Although there is limited documentation of the specific effectiveness of treatment, and treatment selection tends to be based on personal preference and experience rather than on replicable studies of procedures (Pattison, 1977), both authors believe that a chemically dependent nurse, especially one whose addiction has led to professional confrontation, needs intensive treatment.

Stages of Recovery

Detoxification

The first phase of treatment for chemical dependency has as its goal the physiological removal of the substance from the body and the establishment of biochemical equilibrium subsequent to withdrawal.

Assessment factors include:

1. addictive substance(s) used;
2. frequency and quantity of ingestion;
3. last (most recent) use;
4. general physical health;
5. history of previous withdrawals including signs, symptoms, duration;
6. general psychological status, i.e., evidence of hallucinations, agitation, depression, suicidal ideation; and

7. social support systems, such as those with whom the nurse lives, and significant others.

Entry into treatment for chemical dependency is prompted by a crisis—some event or series of events has convinced the nurse that help must be sought. This recognition may be as superficial as agreeing to seek help to get others "off my back." On the other hand, the nurse may acknowledge the addiction to be life threatening. In either event, the prospect of not having access to the chemical substance of choice is frightening and anxiety producing. This thought alone may trigger intense craving for the substance. Often, knowing the "rules" of acceptable behavior in the health care system, the nurse is unlikely to reveal these feelings to health care providers. As a result, even in the initial intake interviews the nurse may knowingly withhold information. The extent to which the nurse is *aware* of providing incomplete or inaccurate information will partly be a function of the nurse's physical condition.

The idea that a specific course of detoxification can be anticipated is probably a myth. As a general rule, heath care providers can expect withdrawal from a chemical substance to produce the opposite effects of the drug. Onset of withdrawal symptoms is dependent on the chemical used.

Signs and symptoms, common to withdrawal from alcohol, narcotics, and sedatives/hypnotics include nausea, vomiting, diaphoresis, insomnia, headache, weakness, apprehension, and irritability. These same signs and symptoms may be seen in tranquilizer withdrawal, although in the case of diazepam (Valium®) the symptoms are delayed in onset. Symptoms of Valium withdrawal peak between the fifth and ninth abstinent day. It is particularly important in known or suspected cross-addictions that in the detoxification process, care providers be alert to differential withdrawal rates. For example, there is some evidence that alcoholics self-medicate for hangover with Valium and develop physical dependence on Valium as well. In such cases, symptoms of alcohol withdrawal would be expected to occur in the first 24 to 72 hours following cessation of drug intake. In the subsequent 72 to 96 hours these symptoms could recur reflecting the withdrawal from Valium.

The specific therapeutic aims during the detoxification phase are to protect the person from complications of withdrawal and to minimize discomfort. The in-patient settings in which this care is provided range from intensive care units to detoxification areas on chemical dependency units. The management of detoxification in an in-patient setting is mandated in the following circumstances of chemical dependence:

1. history of delirium tremens or convulsions in previous withdrawal;
2. extreme agitation, depression or suicidal ideation;
3. heavy alcohol ingestion (fifth/gallon daily) for an extended period;
4. hallucinations, hypo/hypertension, extreme tremulousness.

In addition to these physical/psychological symptoms mandating in-patient detoxification, such placement is also warranted when the overall resources of the client are assessed as inadequate to the maintenance of abstinence.

Generally speaking, there are two primary approaches to the in-patient management of the symptoms of withdrawal. One approach is labeled medical management and in this context refers to the administration of some medication. Tranquilizers are administered in dosages that taper on a daily basis. The intent is to minimize discomfort of withdrawal at a level of dosage low enough to preclude manifestation of the symptoms of the drug (lethargy, disengagement). The other approach is referred to as social detoxification and entails no medication. The interventions include comfort measures, controlled environment, and support. These provisions are most commonly described as: quiet room with subdued lighting, caring management of untoward symptoms, and the presence of others with whom the withdrawing person can talk. There has been some investigation of the relative efficacy of these two approaches in the management of withdrawal symptoms in detoxification. Although the results of such studies remain inconclusive, there is some evidence to suggest that the greater the withdrawing individual's comfort (controlled symptoms) during detoxification, the higher the commitment to recovery as manifested by compliance with a treatment regimen (Gorelick & Wilkins, 1986). On the basis of this finding, it seems that medication should be provided as symptoms indicate.

Nurses presenting for assessment have usually been confronted by significant others directly or indirectly. This confrontation may have occurred within a professional context in which some ultimatum was given—"You must get treatment or lose your license to practice nursing—lose your job, etc." The intervention may have occurred within family context—"If you don't sober up, I'm getting a divorce —or taking the children—or throwing you out." Or, the realization of the seriousness of the problem may have been a personal discovery —"I can't go on like this." In any event, the nurse presenting will be in crisis and, if not intoxicated or high, will likely be physically ill—nauseated, diaphoretic, shaky, aware of tachycardia. In the overwhelming majority of cases the chemically dependent person entering treatment will be moderately to severely depressed, remorseful, and experience profound shame and guilt. These psychological reactions are more intensely experienced by women because of the stereotyping of addiction and labeling of female alcoholics and addicts.

A discussion of the stigma associated with chemically dependent women is beyond the scope of this chapter. Nonetheless, since the overwhelming majority of addicted nurses are women, it seems relevant to digress briefly.

The process of "stigmatization" in the addictive diseases has been documented (Volinn, 1983). In fact, it is only in recent years that chemical dependency has been viewed as an illness as opposed to an intrinsic "badness" in the afflicted person (Conrad & Schneider, 1980). To date, the bulk of research on chemical dependency has used predominately male samples. Although efforts are underway to explore systematically the gender specific differences in chemical dependency, much remains unknown. Despite these caveats, it seems clear that a double standard prevails in our society regarding addiction (Gomberg, 1976), some of which relates to the effect of substance abuse during childbearing years. Women are generally purported to display more affective disorders than men on intake to treatment and suffer from lower self-esteem (Beckman et al., 1980).

It appears as if the behaviors generally associated with a chemically "high" person, such as promiscuity and raucousness, are more acceptable in men than women. Further, the absence from the home for time "on the town" is discouraged for mothers, yet tolerated for fathers. These gender distinctions in society as a whole may be the reason that the "spoiled identity" (Goffman, 1963) of the female addict is more deeply experienced.

A married woman with children may experience intense ambivalence about treatment: although she may recognize treatment as essential to the maintenance of the marriage and/or the appropriate care of her children, she may be unable to envision how she can enter treatment and simultaneously manage the demands in her family life.

In addition to the conflicts they experience over family responsibilities, nurses whose addiction has affected their professional practice may be demoralized by the failure to fulfill professional responsibilities and the violation of the standards and ethics of their professions.

In-patient detoxification can minimize side effects, offer speedy intervention in the event of escalation of symptoms, and provide a controlled environment that can minimize the nurse's discomfort. Almost equally as important as these physical advantages of in-patient detoxification are numerous psychological and social advantages. First, the nurse will be in a setting in which it will be very difficult, if not impossible, to procure the drug of choice, an alternative chemical, or a substance to assuage craving. Second, the nurse will be removed from the family and/or social context that stimulated, protected, or provided for the addiction. Finally, the nurse will be in an environment with persons (detoxifying health professionals or others) who are either experiencing comparable feelings or who have recently experienced them.

These newly abstinent patients provide considerable support to other patients in detoxification and can also provide encouragement regarding the relatively short duration, in most cases, of acute withdrawal symptoms.

The authors believe that in most instances detoxification for chemically-impaired nurses should occur in an in-patient setting. In addition to the advantages of in-patient detoxification discussed above, which are applicable to all chemically impaired people, nurses have some unique needs that may require intense in-patient intervention. An important factor may be the knowledge that the nurse possesses about addiction. In this instance, the knowledge may be a "dangerous thing." Historically, nursing educators have taught students about addiction using the model of psychopathology, i.e., individuals drink excessively or use drugs abusively because of some underlying pathological psychodynamic. As a result, addicted nurses will search obsessively within themselves to discern why they drink and/or use drugs. Nurses (and other health care professionals) must "unlearn" some erroneous assumptions before they can recognize that addiction is a primary disease entity. This process is best begun during the crisis phases of abstinence when denial and rationalization are not as strong and the individual is vulnerable, if not open to new learning. Concentrated contact with health care providers and other chemically dependent clients offers expanded opportunity for this learning to occur.

Another aspect of the nurse's professional socialization best addressed in an in-patient setting is the nurse's sense of responsibility for the nurturing of others. Because they provide comfort and care to others in their professional lives (and often extensively in their personal lives, as well), nurses are uncomfortable accepting help from others. The in-patient environment clearly casts the impaired nurse in the patient role and overtly requires the acceptance of care from others. The in-patient setting also facilitates confrontation of the nurse who has extreme difficulty being in a dependent-patient role. Interventions of this kind may engage the nurse in the therapeutic process during the crisis period of detoxification.

Although every effort should be made to place the chemically dependent nurse in an in-patient setting for detoxification, there are some situations in which this will not be possible. Willingness to undergo assessment at a treatment facility does not mean that the nurse is ready to follow recommendations. The nurse may continue to rationalize the chemical dependence, most commonly at this juncture through the defense mechanism of minimization. In this process, the nurse may admit to abuse of a substance but deny dependence, perhaps belligerently and defiantly. The treatment team then needs to determine if they will attempt some intervention on an out-patient basis or try some compromise with the client.

Management of belligerence and defiance during assessment requires considerable patience and sensitivity. This behavior, commonly associated with the stereotype of the alcoholic or drug addict, should be viewed as a simple attempt on the part of a frightened, physically ill person in crisis to hold onto a familiar way of life regardless of how dysfunctional or self-destructive it may appear to others.

Experts in addiction disagree on the appropriate response in this situation. Some take the position that a person demonstrating this behavior is not ready for treatment, or in the words of Alcoholics Anonymous—has not "hit bottom." This term describes the situation in which the addicted person has lost so much — family, friends, professional standing, financial resources — that denial of the situation's severity is no longer possible. Although hitting bottom is relative and highly individualized, some experts believe that it is a prerequisite to meaningful treatment. When evidence of hitting bottom is lacking, the chemically dependent person may be so advised and told to return for treatment when ready.

Another viewpoint is that any treatment is better than no treatment. In this view, although improvement will sometimes fall short of optimum recovery, every attempt should be made to foster treatment of the addiction. If the nurse agrees only to return in a few days for a check-up, this should be accepted. The rationale here is that at least a link has been established.

Another situation all too common for the chemically dependent woman is an inability to enter in-patient treatment because of child-care responsibilities. If one holds the view that these responsibilities themselves play a role in the addiction, other care-takers in the nurse's family/social network or social service agencies must be sought for child care. This latter option is usually abhorrent to the nurse, as functioning in the parent role might remain one area of continued competence. If no other options exist, careful plans should be made for detoxification on an out-patient basis.

Initial Sobriety

For the purposes of this chapter, initial sobriety has been defined as the first week to ten days after detoxification. We believe that this time after detoxification is of crucial importance, for it is during this period that the individual decides whether or not to continue treatment without the influence of mind-altering substances.

Nurses who have worked on Medical–Surgical units and cared for patients in acute delirium tremens may be familiar with the following scenario. The patient appears to have suffered extensively in withdrawal. The symptoms abate and the patient is prepared for discharge with information as to the dire consequences of a return to drinking or using drugs. The patient swears "never again" and in apparent good spirits leaves the hospital. Yet, in a week, the health care team finds the patient readmitted in the same state. Or worse, the team learns that the patient has died. This scenario occurs because the behavior of initial sobriety has not been understood and the client was discharged in the most dangerous stage of recovery.

What appears to occur is that as the acute withdrawal symptoms subside and the crisis of the confrontation necessitating treatment begins to resolve, the individual resurrects the defenses of minimization and rationalization. Concurrently, as the physical manifestations of withdraw lessen, the patient begins to feel better than at any time in recent memory. The convergence of these forces leads to the patient's being in "good spirits," and the old justifications return to the thinking. Denial returns and is established on physical evidence (feeling good). As a result, the patient begins to believe that the situation "wasn't *that* bad" and "how can *one* drink/snort/hit/etc. hurt."

In treating the impaired nurse, it is critical at this juncture that the treatment team emphasize the struggle of detoxification and the factors that brought the nurse to treatment. This tends to be more easily accomplished in an in-patient setting where the patient moves directly from the detoxification to the primary treatment arena. It is very difficult to approach a patient—recently in withdrawal and now cheerful—with the goal of dispelling this cheer and forcing the nurse to experience *emotionally* the plight of chemical dependence. In any treatment setting, the treatment team finds this goal in conflict with their desire to ease the patient's suffering and to see improvement. In an out-patient setting this goal is even more difficult to achieve. The patient can leave the treatment center and return to an environment in which relief from despair and sadness through the use of chemicals is readily available. As a result, the treatment team may be less confronting in an out-patient setting since they are more "fearful" of relapse or treatment drop-out.

Another factor in assessing the treatment needs of the chemically impaired nurse relates to the difficulty nurses have taking care of themselves. By psychosocial predisposition and formal training, they have a strong need to take care of others and avoid caring for themselves. The nurse seems to develop an attitude of "I can handle it" and feel that to admit weakness or inadequacy is dangerous to the well-being of other people. The nurse's limited ability to recognize chemical dependency as a disease requiring the help of others is compounded by an apparent belief that patients are "weak and dependent," the antithesis of the nurse's desired self-perception.

In-patient treatment appears to have an advantage over out-patient treatment in helping the nurse learn how to be a patient with needs, who must follow instructions to meet those needs—in short, to become teachable. Since education of the chemically-dependent person is a large component of the treatment process, this factor is important. The in-patient format allows the patient to talk and "live" addiction and recovery without distractions. Patients receive considerable information and have the opportunity to process it in concert with other people who are also in the learner role.

In learning about cross-addiction, patients can share their experiences and affirm new viewpoints. They learn nonchemical ways of coping and in an in-patient setting have extensive opportunity to practice these skills as they become oriented and develop an understanding of a 12-step program such as Alcoholics Anonymous or Narcotics Anonymous. For example, the spiritual aspects of a recovery program are often difficult for individuals who have negative feelings about early religious experiences and training. Living in a community with others who are struggling to separate their ideas about religion from the spiritual components of the program appears to foster internalization and personalization of spirituality.

In-patient treatment further allows the impaired nurse the opportunity to be removed from the professional arena and the day-to-day stresses associated with responsibilities in multiple roles. Frequently these nurses need time out from the traumas resulting from their disease. Although there are often overwhelming financial, legal, professional, and family problems, the impaired nurse needs a safe place and time for healing to begin. Some persons perceive the expectations of others for their recovery to be overwhelming, so they require physical separation in order to focus on their own healing.

The disadvantages of in-patient treatment in this phase is a mirror reflection of the advantages of out-patient intervention. Although the in-patient environment is safe, it is also artificial (Schukit, 1985) and incongruous with the "real" world. The real world is not a safe place for the chemically dependent person, as it is fraught with many temptations and triggers to use alcohol or drugs. Learning about this aspect and other dimensions of the disease on an out-patient basis may facilitate integration of new information into an existing lifestyle. The assessment skills of the treatment team working in concert with the honest self-appraisals of the nurse can determine the best course of action in each case.

Transition

The period of time following detoxification and the initial period of sobriety, about two weeks subsequent to intervention, has herein been labeled transition. Biochemically, "the fog" of drugs or alcohol has lifted. The nurse physically feels better, is eating normally, and appears sober. Psychologically, the extreme mood swings of the first two weeks have abated somewhat and the nurse has begun to negotiate with "others."

A common behavior during this time is resistance, which is manifested by defiance and hostile outbursts toward the treatment team. Some authorities speculate that the real resistance is not to treatment but to abstinence. A therapeutic intervention found to be effective in countering this resistance, regardless of the site of treatment, is group therapy. It is believed that the intense transference occurring in the therapeutic relationship is reflected in resistance and outbursts of hostility (Zimberg, 1982). Group therapy has been found to be an effective way of diffusing this transference.

One explanation of the diffusion of transference may lie in the unconditional acceptance that appears to prevail in therapeutic groups. The person is accepted by the group *no matter* what has occurred in the past. This environment stands in marked contrast to the multiple demands with many recriminations that the addict in early recovery must face in other arenas.

Another important function of therapeutic groups relates to the domain of feelings. Chemically dependent people are generally out of touch with their feelings; in fact, chemical dependency may be viewed as a disease of altered feelings. As addiction progresses, addicts, particularly women, tend to isolate themselves. Their relationships become increasingly superficial and they are able to share less and less of themselves. It is not uncommon to see chemically impaired nurses in treatment who have not experienced a genuine feeling in years. Although they appear angry and frightened, these feelings seem symptomatic of the fears and pathology surrounding their drug or alcohol use. Within a therapeutic group, the nurse begins to explore feelings, to recognize and label different emotions. The group further serves the important function of validating and affirming the feelings expressed by a person who is very vulnerable.

Experience in the group also helps the recovering person to develop the ability to confront others about important issues. Nurses, predominantly women, have not generally been taught to confront each other, and many find themselves caught in a conspiracy of silence. Although this seems especially true regarding the use of alcohol or drugs in the professional arena, it is no less true with regard to other aspects of intraprofessional relationships.

Therapeutic groups are particularly important in confronting denial: the denial is caused by the alterations in perception occasioned by the chemical, and the denial of the severe psychic pain that may have preceded, but definitely follows, chemical dependence. It seems to be very difficult for nurses to turn control over to others in the way required by groups in a therapeutic setting. The fear of being powerless is unacceptable to most nurses, as is the fear of not being able to manage their own lives. Nurses seem to believe that if they are not in control of themselves, all the people around them will not survive. The most painful aspect of treatment to them is not the divorce or the loss of a job, money, etc., but being confronted with the fact that they are not in control and may not have been for some time. The realization of the truth of this insight produces a loss of personal respect and exquisite pain. The recovering nurse needs a safe, protective, and supportive environment to confront these truths.

Clearly, intensive group therapy can occur on an out-patient basis. The advantage of in-patient therapy is the continuous and contiguous involvement with the same group of people. Relationships are established outside the context of the therapy sessions, and the recovering individuals share in the same community.

Depending on the organization of the treatment program, out-patient groups can be very effective. At the present time there is a general questioning of the expensive in-patient approaches (Moore, 1977), particularly in the face of limited data to substantiate systematically that outcomes between the two approaches differ. There is some evidence that the drop-out rate from treatment is higher in out-patient programs than in-patient (Baekeland, 1977). It may well be that out-patient programs do not engage the addict as effectively in the treatment process or maximize motivation toward abstinence, which Schukit (1985) claims as the raison d'être of in-patient approaches.

Early Recovery

As the impaired nurse enters early recovery, the issues of reentry loom large in treatment planning. It is in this phase of recovery that some of the advantages of intense out-patient treatment can become more evident. Within that format, the nurse has been maintaining some relationships and has begun to make assessments of lifestyle based on daily attempts to integrate the learning experiences of treatment into previous patterns. The ongoing feedback from group therapy has assisted in clarifying problems and identifying sources of support to use in decision making.

The nurse who has received treatment in an in-patient setting has been protected from many of the assaults to sobriety that the out-patient nurse has experienced. At the same time, however, this individual has not had the opportunity to practice new skills or apply new understanding in "real" situations. As discharge from the in-patient setting approaches, this nurse must confront and manage separation anxiety and develop anticipatory strategies to deal with stressful events that in the past were dealt with chemically. After a month or so in a chemically-free environment, the nurse must marshall the resources to combat anew the ready accessibility of chemicals. This is a dimension of recovery that the out-patient treatment modality has incorporated on a continuous basis and that the nurse, successfully treated in that format, has begun to integrate as an ongoing mode of operation.

Both authors believe that nurses need intense treatment to prepare themselves for the "fallout" of their disease. The misperceptions that prevail in the general public are rampant within the profession as well, and the recovering person must be prepared to deal with the rejection of persons who have been stigmatized. At home, at work, and in multiple relationships, the newly recovering person will not be trusted. Role playing within the group context is helpful in assisting the impaired nurse to anticipate these responses from others and to develop methods of dealing with them. Many nurses in early recovery report feelings bordering on paranoia, although the perceptions of the recovering person are frequently very accurate: colleagues, friends, and family tend to anticipate relapse. Irritability or short temperedness, common behaviors in persons adapting to new roles, are viewed by others as symptomatic of imminent or actual return to drinking or using other drugs.

Although the intensity of treatment (generally considered as synonymous with in-patient treatment) may be a source of relief to some people in the lives of the impaired nurse, the reverse might be equally true. For example, one supervisor of an impaired nurse, who is about to return to work after treatment, may believe that the intense treatment assures the recovery of the nurse, whereas another supervisor might believe that the very intensity reflects the severity of the nurse's addiction, causing little reason to expect continued sobriety. The possibility that these two disparate beliefs might be held about the same nurse demonstrates the world of mixed messages and conflicting expectations that the nurse in early recovery experiences.

An important dimension in the continuum of care that addresses these and other adjustment issues is aftercare. Treatment of the impaired nurse following primary care must be planned to assist the in-patient client to make the transition of reentry and to provide ongoing support and help to the nurse in early recovery. The goals of aftercare are to facilitate reentry to various roles and occupations while simultaneously consolidating gains in personal growth made in treatment (Gitlow & Peyser, 1980).

Aftercare provides the nurse with continued relationships within the treatment agency and with members of their patient therapeutic groups. Aftercare groups of recovering health professionals can be particularly helpful to each other as they deal with issues of returning to a work-a-day world fraught with stresses and easy accessibility to drugs-of-choice and alcohol.

Frequently, it is in aftercare when the full impact of the effects of the addiction will "hit" the impaired nurse. The financial chaos, the broken marriage, the lost job and/or license to practice, the acting out children, the rejecting parents — the list could be endless. Extending the effect of treatment through a comprehensive aftercare program can assist the impaired nurse in early recovery to deal with these problems in a constructive, responsible, and chemically free manner.

Ongoing Recovery

Since recovery from addiction is ongoing, efforts to maintain sobriety must become part of the daily life of the impaired nurse. Consistent participation in a 12-step recovery program and careful attention to the HALT warning (*H*ungry, *A*ngry, *L*onely, *T*ired) of personal indicators of stress can lead to continuous sobriety. Solid recovery is commonly recognized after two years of uninterrupted sobriety with reasonable satisfaction in adjustment. During ongoing recovery, it is hoped that the impaired nurse will find increased satisfaction in work and life and continue with personal and professional growth.

References

Baekeland, F., & Lundwall, L. (1977). Dropping out of treatment: A critical review. *Psychological Bulletin, 82*(5), 738–783.

Beckman, L., Day, T., Bardsley, P., & Seeman, A. (1980). The personality characteristics and family background of women alcoholics. *International Journal of Addictions, 15,* 147–154.

Brown, S. (1985). *Treating the alcoholic: A developmental model of recovery.* New York: Wiley.

Conrad, P., & Schneider, J. W. (1980). *Deviance and medicalization, from badness to sickness.* St. Louis, MO: Mosby.

Gitlow, S. E., & Reyser, H. S. (Eds.). (1980). *Alcoholism: A practical treatment guide.* New York: Grune & Stratton.

Goffman, E. (1963). *Stigma: Notes on the management of a spoiled identity.* Englewood Cliffs, NJ: Prentice Hall.

Gomberg, E. (1976). The female alcoholic. In R. Tarter & A. Sugarmen (Eds.). *Alcoholism: interdisciplinary approaches to an enduring problem* (pp. 603–620). Reading, MA: Addison-Wesley.

Gorelick, D. A., & Wilkins, J. N. (1986). Special aspects of human alcohol withdrawal. In M. Galanter (Ed.), *Recent developments in alcoholism: Vol. 4* (pp. 283–305). New York: Alenum Press.

Moore, L. (1977) Ten years of in-patient programs for alcoholic patients. *American Journal of Psychiatry, 134*(5), 542–545.

Pattison, E. M. (1977). Ten years of change in alcoholism treatment and delivery. *American Journal of Psychiatry, 134*(3), 261–266.

Schuckit, M. A. (1985). Inpatient and residential approaches to the treatment of alcoholism. In J. H. Mundelson & N. K. Mello (Eds.). *Diagnosis and treatment of alcoholism* (pp. 325–354). New York: McGraw Hill.

Volinn, I. (1983). Health professionals as stigmatizers and destigmatizers of diseases: Alcoholism and leprosy as examples. *Social Science and Medicine, 17,* 385–393.

Zimberg, S. (1982). *The clinical management of alcoholism.* New York: Brunner/Mazel.

7

Intervention with Nurses in Academia and Administration

Beverly J. McElmurry, Olga M. Church, and Mary R. Haack

This chapter discusses chemical impairment among nurses who hold administrative or faculty positions in the clinical or academic arena. While it is recognized that not all of these positions are held by women, the focus of this discussion is on the difficulties associated with recognizing chemical impairment among female nurses holding upper level management or faculty positions and with determining appropriate interventions in such situations.

Recognizing Chemical Impairment in Nursing Leaders

Scope of the Problem

Examining society's views and expectations of women is critical to any consideration of chemical impairment among women. Furthermore, in addition to social factors, physiologic differences between men and women must be considered when examining the effects of alcohol and other drugs on the body. Within the past decade, research on occupational alcoholism has illuminated some of the problems inherent in chemical dependence in the work place. Yet studies specific to employees in management positions are few.

In general, "research indicates that certain characteristics of management jobs—such as freedom to set one's own work hours, frequent assignments outside the work setting, and low interdependence with other jobs in the organization—permit managers to cover up their impairment while on the job and to avoid high rates of absenteeism" (Kleeman & Googins, 1983, p. 22).

A faculty member has similar working conditions (McMillan, 1985). Thoreson (1984) cogently describes alcohol abuse in academe and suggests that "characteristics of academics and academe intertwine to produce an ecological system that is, paradoxically, ideally constructed to nurture both the wellspring of creativity requisite to a community of scholars and the development of alcohol abuse" (p. 56). The academician, in Thoreson's view, is "barely supervised and basically unsupervisable" (p. 63).

It is estimated that in the general population 70% of the people drink. Of those who drink, approximately 10% of the men and 5% of the women drinkers are estimated to be problem drinkers (U.S. Department of Health and Human Services, 1987). One can use the most recent Sigma Theta Tau Directory of Nurse Researchers (Barnard, Kiener, & Fawcett, 1987) to estimate the prevalence of alcoholism in a group that represents a nursing leadership component. The Directory lists a total of 3,681 researchers; if 70% or 2,577 of them drink, perhaps 5% or 129 of them have a serious problem. Another example can be drawn from the National League for Nursing (1986) listing of 8,944 full-time faculty in baccalaureate and higher degree programs. Again, if 70% drink (6,261) and 5% have a problem, there is a possibility that 313 are alcoholics. Given what we expect of these groups professionally and the extensive preparation required to become an active researcher or educator, it is obvious how important and serious this problem is for a profession such as nursing.

Within the past decade, concerns about alcohol in the work place have been examined by the collection of surveys on the prevalence of drinking within specific occupational populations, as well as the characteristics of occupations. Studies of occupational status as related to drinking behavior have identified the factors of time pressure and job stress as worthy of further investigation.

According to Pearlin (1982), it is useful to distinguish when the work place is either a primary source of drinking problems, a reinforcing source, or a domain of experience that has little or nothing to do with drinking. Acknowledging the importance of the work role in our society, conditions that shape work and regulate experiences on the job are significant (Pearlin, 1982, p. 130). If, in fact, negative experiences related to stress or other factors contribute to the "professional problem," then the work place serves as a paradox. That is, it may not only serve as a contributing source of the problem, but at the same time prevent the employee or faculty member as described by Thoreson from coping with the working environment. As Pearlin (1982) points out, intervention within the working environment may well be limited to the extent that "the very authority system that is enlisted to force the worker into treatment may also be a contributor to his or her drinking problem" (p. 132).

During the past decade, occupational alcoholism has become a subject for investigation. Surveys and studies related to women and alcohol have begun to emerge. Not surprisingly, the professional literature reveals a discernible movement toward self-scrutiny in nursing during this same period. Given the predominance of women in the field of nursing, it is also pertinent to note that employed women have a higher rate of alcoholism than unemployed women. This may be the consequence of the liberation of women's roles. More women drink now, therefore, more women develop dependence. Among women who are alcoholic, a significantly increased risk of abuse of prescribed drugs exists.

According to Solomon (1984), many high achieving women are burdened with dual time demands and responsibilities for both home and career. Those who do not opt for marriage and family risk facing pressures imposed by a family-oriented society. Women with children have additional responsibilities to manage, and single parents enjoy less support and must cope with the pressure of seeking companionship and love relationships. Role strain was a significant factor reported by the academic nurses in Gerace's doctoral dissertation (1987).

Imes and Clance (1984) postulate that high achieving women often believe they are frauds and not as bright, capable, or creative as the evidence would support. These women are secretly convinced that they have fooled everyone and live in fear that they will be found out. How these women cope with such conflict is an important question. Since many administrative and academic nurses function autonomously, oftentimes without significant interaction with peers, the coping strategies used by this group may also be solitary in nature. Drinking or taking drugs can be a very private activity which numbs the feelings of inadequacy and loneliness.

At the managerial level, chemical dependency becomes a delicate issue, for the risk of exposure is a constant threat, and the higher up the echelon, the harder the fall. The nature of leadership implies seasoned wisdom and intellectual awareness, yet the nature of drug/chemical dependency implies loss of control and awareness and lost credibility.

As a predominately female profession, nurses and nursing are viewed in large part the way all women are viewed. The changing status of women, especially during the past decade, has profoundly affected the nursing profession (ANA, 1984). This altered status is reflected by the emerging research on women in our society.

Examination of alcohol problems in women managers raises the question of whether alcoholic women in management might be in jeopardy of losing their jobs or denied promotions. Data on employee assistance programs (EAPs) reveal that managers are underrepresented as program participants. In particular, there has been a dearth of data on impaired female employees in management positions. It may be that the EAP model is not the most effective way to help the nurse manager, or it is possible that female alcoholic managers are fired before assistance from an EAP is sought.

While some progress has been made since the conspiracy of silence was officially broken by the ANA resolution in 1982, nurses whose functioning is impaired by alcohol or drugs continue to be stigmatized. Substance dependence carries a stereotypic stigma that, not unlike sexism, racism, and ageism, for the most part, prevents it from being viewed seriously as an illness worthy of active intervention and treatment. This lack of knowledge about the illness and its ramifications is pervasive—both within and outside of the profession. Even those of our colleagues who recognize substance dependence as an illness commonly enter into the conspiracy of silence rather than risk retribution by confronting the reality and dealing with it.

It has been said that the nursing profession has traditionally reacted like a dysfunctional family in regard to the chemically dependent members of our professional family (Haack, 1986, p. 688). That is, "we deny, we protect, we accept excuses, we try to ignore the problem and hope it will go away and, finally, we fire or jerk the license and pitch them out" (Green, 1983, p. 18).

Identifying the Impaired Nurse Leader

Who is to say that a nurse leader is chemically impaired? We hope that it is someone who cares about the person. More often than not, however, the problem is brought to the attention of nursing colleagues by others, such as faculty and friends outside the work setting, who have not been able to help the person with the problem. Job performance is usually the last to be affected by chemical dependency. If the leader is a colleague and lines of authority and power are insignificant, discussing one's concern with them will not seem difficult. However, confronting a nurse leader is a situation of potential risk, especially to a subordinate. By virtue of the leadership position, a nurse whose functioning is impaired can occupy an untouchable position. Such positions, paradoxically, are characterized by interpersonal isolation.

Enabling

Once the existence of a substance-dependence problem in a nurse leader, has been established colleagues and superiors must examine what role they play in its continuance. One can either be part of the solution or part of the problem, i.e., an enabler. What is an enabler? It is anyone who compensates for the lapses observed in an impaired co-worker's performance. Most of us have been enablers. Most of the time we were or are unwitting enablers. We expect others to be rational and to control drinking or drug use. We believe the colleague who promises to seek help, or we accept attempts at seeking help from psychotherapists or family doctors who do not address the substance-dependence problem. We justify the drinking or drug use: "Her job put her under a lot of pressure." We protect the person's image by hiring competent and supportive secretarial help. We allow subordinates to take over responsibilities that belong to the administrator or professor. We are enablers because of ignorance and coverups. The fact is that we often fail to assess and identify alcohol as the problem or even to consider the potential of substance dependence as a problem when we educate and socialize people as health care professionals. We teach about mood-altering and pain-relieving substances but we seldom teach nonchemical ways of relieving pain or stress symptoms. In addition, very few nurses have received any formal education in substance abuse.

Hoffman and Heinemann (1987) conducted a national survey in 1,035 nursing schools on substance abuse education. Of the 336 schools of nursing that responded, 72% reported one to five hr of required instruction in substance abuse illness. (It is important to note that most baccalaureate programs in nursing have more than 800 clinical hr and 350 didactic hr of nursing content.) Disturbingly, the study's findings demonstrated very little, if any, clinical experience with clients who were receiving treatment for their alcohol and substance abuse problems.

A historical review of the professional nursing literature which examined the content that identified alcohol and drug consumption in general, and in relationship to the nurse or nursing in particular, revealed glimpses of concern. However, by design or default, during the first eight decades of this century, the professional nursing literature indicates a collective denial or conspiracy of silence on the subject, especially as it related to nurses or nursing in particular (Church, 1985).

The care of clients with addictions as a legitimate area of nursing practice has only recently been recognized by the American Nurses' Association (ANA, 1987). The ANA has also provided the profession with parameters defining nursing's responsibilities and standards within the chemical dependency specialty (ANA, 1987). Referring to this specialty as "Addictions Nursing," the ANA acknowledges the relatively recent emergence of this special area of nursing care and bases the parameters of practice on the premise that "human beings have an inherent capacity for change and actualization toward health" (ANA, 1987). Given that the study of substance abuse disorders has been limited to a small group within the profession, it is not surprising that nurses do not know how to help a colleague who is impaired.

Response to and Interventions with the Chemically Impaired Nurse Leader

The following imaginary dialogue is an exchange between subordinates as they discuss their supervisor.

> "What should we do? If we arrange an intervention, will it work? What if she refuses to enter treatment and instead sues us for infringing on her rights, questioning her competence or damaging her reputation? It's none of our business! But, you can see that she is suffering; her color is poor, she looks bloated and there has been a personality change. Dealing with her is more and more difficult! You can't just stand by and watch her destroy herself. But, we have no proof that she is an alcoholic. Yes, but everyone says that they smell alcohol on her breath. Well, if I were you, I'd keep out of other people's business. What's it to you anyway?"

Anyone who has agonized over what to do about an impaired co-worker has heard some of the above comments. Any reader of this chapter who has wondered, as we have, about what to do when a co-worker is obviously chemically impaired understands why we are writing. It is not easy to watch someone self-destruct. The authors have experienced the loss of notable colleagues to addiction-related deaths. These are not just personal losses, but losses to the profession.

Many nurse leaders are nursing scholars who are of significant value to the profession and society. When these leaders suffer, because of the problems caused by their substance dependency, the profession suffers. Dorsey and Scheer (1987) make an important point in their discussion of the licensing board's treatment of substance dependent professionals. That is, the overriding purpose of confrontation and intervention with chemically impaired colleagues is to balance public protection with support for individual rehabilitation. This view would also be consistent with Fowler (1986) and Naegle's (1985) discussions of our ethical responsibilities to both colleagues and patients.

Once impairment is identified in a colleague, what are the options? First of all, there is limited information available about approaches that work. There are some reports of training nurses in confrontational strategies. For example, Finke (1986) reported that nurses who were taught how to confront the problem drinker subsequently made more interventions than a comparison group without such preparation. O'Connor and Robinson (1985) urged administrators to focus their initial efforts in dealing with a problem employee on the staff's enabling behavior. It is important to encourage a work environment where trust and open communication is the norm. Yet the early identification and intervention with chemically dependent women is unlikely because the social taboos against addiction in women delay the recognition and treatment of this disease (Rachel, 1985).

The recent articles about Betty Ford and her family (Ford & Chase, 1987) and the work of Vernon Johnson (1986) have made the use of "intervention" more visible to the public. This method, which we favor, involves a group of people who care about the chemically dependent person. Group members plan and conduct a confrontation in which they each explain how the person's drinking is affecting them. The emphasis in such confrontations is that the people who organize it genuinely care about the person and want to help. There is rightful concern that the form of intervention described is designed for a middle-class group. In our experience, most nursing leaders with a drinking problem fall into this socioeconomic category.

A major consideration in any intervention with a chemically dependent person is preplanning. We have used our experience to identify some questions that need to be considered:

- Is there a colleague with expertise (an alcohol counselor/nurse psychotherapist) available to guide the people considering a confrontation?
- Will the employee's professional or personal insurance cover treatment for substance dependence?

- Will the immediate supervisor of the person to be confronted support your intervention and make plans for the person's job to be performed by someone else?
- Who will participate in the confrontation?
- Who in the work environment knows the family and whether or not the family is likely to go along with the plan? Or, should the family be left out of the intervention?
- If the family is not included in the confrontation, who will inform them that the intervention has taken place?
- If the person is to go from the confrontation to an assessment or treatment facility, how will you decide which one?
- What treatment facilities have experience and expertise in dealing with chemically dependent professionals, especially chemically dependent women?
- Are there means for ensuring that the nurse's responsibilities at home are covered, e.g., care of children, or elderly parents?
- Who will accompany the nurse to the assessment or treatment setting after the confrontation?
- What will others in the work setting be told about the intervention prior to or after its implementation?
- How do colleagues and co-workers demonstrate their caring and supportive behaviors when a person is in treatment?
- What can colleagues do to ensure a successful return to work after treatment?
- Upon return to work how can colleagues demonstrate patience and acceptance of the recovering nurse as she develops new relationships with colleagues?

The initial confrontation or reaching out to an impaired colleague may be informal and on a one-to-one basis. It should always be done by someone who is a respected peer or authority figure. This can take the form of explicit concern: "I've really been concerned about your drinking" with some discussion of examples for the concern. Ultimately, the informal conversation should get to "I wish you would think about getting help. I will be glad to assist you in that." If this approach fails, a group intervention should be considered. Usually, several informal attempts at helping are made before a formal intervention is planned.

deGarmo, Lynch, and Pecora (1983) note the crisis state precipitated by this type of intervention and offer some useful confrontation guidelines. The points they make and which our experience supports are: (1) Several people should be involved in the intervention, preferably people with a meaningful relationship to the nurse. Ideally, one of the persons will have training in the intervention process. (2) The people who will conduct the intervention should prepare in advance for the intervention. Those to be involved need to meet as a group at least once before the confrontation to clarify the approach and assess their comfort in conducting the intervention. (3) If possible, documented observations of impaired job performance are prepared for presentation during the confrontation. (4) The intervention should be conducted in a caring and firm manner. (5) Suitable and immediately available treatment alternatives should be confirmed before the intervention and these choices presented to the person during the confrontation. (6) All persons involved should be clear that the goal of the intervention is to get the nurse into treatment.

The American Psychological Association has delineated the following six steps in confronting and supporting a distressed colleague (VandenBos & Duthie, 1986). They are appropriate for the nurse leader as well.

Step 1: Evaluate the Information

The first step is to systematically evaluate the available data that generates concern. This involves listing behaviors and events that concern you (being specific to time, place, and detail). If some of the behaviors have been reported by others, consider carefully the credibility of that individual. The impaired functioning of particular concern are: substance abuse related health problems, mood swings, paranoid behavior, inappropriate social behavior, evidence of family violence, telephone calls made at inappropriate times that the person has no memory of, absenteeism or inconsistent work performance, alcohol breath during work hours, and regular use of tranquilizers or sleeping pills. Signs of depression such as unkempt appearance, flat affect, complaints of sleep disturbance, or suicidal ideation can signal a primary affective disorder or a substance abuse induced depression. It is important not to make a diagnosis or label a person an alcoholic. An indepth assessment should be done by a skilled clinician as an outcome of the intervention.

Step 2: Decide Who Should Confront the Individual

The most appropriate people to intervene are peers and/or supervisors who genuinely care about the person. It is also useful to involve significant others such as spouses or children. It is important to assess the enabling potential of both family members and peers. It is not uncommon for an alcoholic nurse to be married to an alcoholic spouse. Alcoholic spouses or colleagues will sabotage an intervention. They should not be included. If the impaired nurse is in therapy at the time, the therapist should be notified and invited to participate in the intervention.

In considering an intervention with an academic or administrative nurse, the issue of position of authority is critical. No subordinate or academic of a lesser rank should attempt an intervention without the active involvement of those in power. Certainly, no student should attempt an intervention with a faculty member. If a subordinate or academic of less rank is skilled in substance abuse treatment he or she may be very useful in the preparation step of the intervention but should probably not be actively involved in the intervention itself.

Step 3: Prepare Before the Meeting

It is important that all people involved in the intervention participate in organizing and discussing what will take place. It is impossible to predict how a nurse leader will respond. It is realistic to expect denial and anger, but it is not uncommon for the individual to express relief. It is important for each person involved in the intervention to express their own fears and reservations in confronting the individual. Most people have a significant amount of ambivalence that needs to be worked through before the intervention is attempted. Discussion of who plays what role also needs to take place during the preparation meeting. All persons should be clear that the goal of intervention is to facilitate the nurse's entry into treatment. Treatment programs especially designed for professionals are ideal.

Suitable treatment alternatives should be confirmed before the intervention takes place.

Step 4: Consider How You Will Address Your Colleague

It is important that a leader be designated who will address the impaired colleague and facilitate participation of all who are present. It is essential to stick to the specifics. Describe succinctly the facts of the behavior you have observed and explain why the behavior is troublesome. Avoid being judgmental or diagnosing. Express understanding, support, and confidence in your colleague's desire to change. An outside consultant may be present to help facilitate the intervention if the group desires this.

Step 5: Speak, Listen, and Discuss

Once all concerns are laid on the table, time to listen and discuss must be allowed. If the person expresses denial and/or anger, allow this to happen and do not become defensive. Continue to be supportive but firm. When the person is able to hear what you are saying, describe the treatment options available. Possible treatment choices should be well researched in advance of the intervention. If none of the suggestions are acceptable, be prepared to set limits. The most powerful limits are an imposed leave of absence or termination of employment. Allow several hours for this step. No one should leave before the step is complete.

Step 6: Follow Up

As soon as the meeting is finished, follow-up on all decisions should be immediate. A thorough assessment should be carried out by a skilled clinician who is at least equal in status to the impaired faculty member or administrator. A diagnostic interview requires a significant amount of self-disclosure which is accomplished more easily if the person feels understood and respected. This is not to say that a very adequate assessment cannot be done by other disciplines or by professionals with fewer degrees. If family members are able to assist the person in preparing for admission to a treatment center, they can take over at this point. If not, someone involved in the intervention should assist the person as needed until he or she is admitted to a treatment program.

In summary, each step of an intervention must be carefully planned. The availability of a person with training in the confrontation process will help the members of the intervention group dispel fears and facilitate the actual intervention. The support of the immediate supervisor is essential. It is important to arrange a referral to a treatment program that will be available for at least two years of treatment follow-up. Ideally, this is a program designed to treat professionals. Overall, careful planning increases the probability of a successful intervention, referral, and recovery.

An intervention with a nurse colleague is an investment of time and resources that can have significant payoff. It can literally save the life of the impaired individual, and it usually has a profound effect on all who are involved in the process. If it is done with thoughtfulness and caring, it brings out the very best in everyone. If it is motivated by a need to punish, the outcome will only add to the many problems the impaired individual must handle in recovery.

The difficulties the person faces when reentering the work environment can be overwhelming. Nurses are socialized to care for people who are ill, but are not taught how to help each other. Often we revert to behavior towards colleagues that we would never tolerate in caring for a patient with a similar problem. We can be insensitive, moralistic, and punitive. It is ironic that profit-oriented corporations such as American Telephone and Telegraph (AT&T), Ford Motor Company, International Business Machines (IBM) all have programs for their employees whose performance is impaired by substance dependence, and none of them terminate or demote an employee who cooperates in seeking and participating in treatment. Yet, it is the norm rather than the exception for nurses who are treated for substance dependence not to return to their former positions. Rather than allowing them the time and resources to recover physically and emotionally, they are often exhorted to prove themselves, a stress that can be destructive in the critical first two years of abstinence.

At the present time, we are unable to identify which nurses are being reached by the existing models of peer assistance or employee assistance. It is our impression that nursing leaders in administration and academe are underserved by the present programs. To our knowledge, no policies exist in schools of nursing or hospitals to guide colleagues in intervening with this population.

Nursing leaders represent a select group which is small in any given setting. It may be unrealistic to expect each university or hospital to have a person or committee trained and skilled in intervention. But it is not unrealistic to expect nurse executive groups to have identified nurses who can advise and facilitate an intervention on a consulting basis.

Nurses in academe and management represent the most educated and influential members of our profession. The time, money, and talent invested in the careers of these individuals are losses nursing can ill afford. The successful intervention with and treatment of these individuals is critical if we are to change attitudes toward the issue of impairment within the profession. If American Airlines, Trans-World Airlines, and United Airlines can support the recovery and maintain the employment status of an impaired pilot, can nursing justify anything less for the leaders of the profession?

References

American Nursing Association. (1984). *Addictions and psychological dysfunctions in nursing: The profession's response to the problem.*Kansas City, MO: Author.

American Nurses' Association and National Nurses Society on Addictions. (1987). *Standards of Addictions Nursing Practice with Selected Diagnoses and Criteria.* Kansas City, MO: American Nurses' Association.

American Nurses' Association and National Nurses Society on Addictions. (1988). *Standards of Addictions Nursing Practice with Selected Diagnoses and Criteria.* Kansas City, MO. American Nurses' Association.

Barnard, R., Kiener, M., & Fawcett, J. (Eds.). (1987). *Directory of Nurse Researchers* (2nd ed.). Indianapolis, IN: Sigma Theta Tau.

Barr, M. A., & Lerner, W. D. (1984). The impaired nurse: A management issue. *Nursing Economics, 2,* 196–201.

Church, O. M. (1985). Sairey Gamp revisited: A historical inquiry into alcoholism and drug dependency. *Nursing Administration Quarterly, 9*(2), 10–21.

deGarmo, P., Lynch, B., & Pecora, V. (1983). Substance abuse: An occupational hazard among nurses (part 3). *Oregon Nurse, 48*(5), 8–9,16,18.

Dorsey, D. M., & Scheer, R. (1987). Licensing boards and impaired professionals. *Maryland Medical Journal, 36*(3), 238–240.

Finke, L. M. (1986). Effect of an educational program on the role of security of medical-surgical nurses towards confronting clients with drinking problems. *Dissertation Abstracts International, 46*(10), 3390–3391 B.

Ford, B., & Chase, C. (1987). *Betty: A glad awakening.* New York: Doubleday.

Fowler, M. D. (1986). Ethical issues in critical care: Doctoring or nursing under the influence. *Heart and Lungs, 15*(2), 205–207.

Gerace, L. (1987). *Role strain: Psychological status and substance use patterns in nurse educators.* Unpublished dissertation, University of Illinois at Chicago, Graduate College.

Green, P. (1983). Chemical dependency in the nursing profession. *Kansas Nurse, 58,* 17–18.

Haack, M. R. (1986). Substance abuse. In B. Logan and C. Dawkins (Eds.), *Family centered nursing in the community* (pp. 669–691). Menlo Park, CA: Addison Wesley.

Hoffman, A. L., & Heinemann, M. E. (1987). Substance abuse education in schools of nursing: A national survey. *Journal of Nursing Education, 26*(7), 282–287.

Imes, S., & Clance, P. R. (1984). Treatment of the imposter phenomenon. In C. M. Brody (Ed.). *Women therapists working with women* (pp. 78–82). New York: Springer.

Jefferson, L. V., & Ensor, B. E. (1982). Help for the helper: Confronting a chemically impaired colleague. *American Journal of Nursing, 82,* 574–577.

Johnson, V. E. (1986). *Intervention: How to help someone who doesn't want help.* Minneapolis, MN: Johnson Institute Books.

Kleeman, B., & Googins, B. (1983). Women alcoholics in management: Issues in identification. *Alcohol Health and Research World, 7*(3), 23–28.

McMillan, L. (1985, October). The alcoholic professor: Campus is ideal environment for a hidden problem. *Chronicle of Higher Education, 9,* 1,26.

Naegle, M. A. (1985). Impaired nursing practice: Ethical and legal issues. *Imprint, 32*(2), 48–53.

National League for Nursing Division of Public Policy and Research. (1986). *Nurse Faculty Socioeconomic Trends, 1985.* New York: NLN.

O'Connor, P., & Robinson, R. S. (1985). Managing impaired nurses. *Nursing Administration Quarterly, 9*(2), 1–9.

Pearlin, L. I. (1982). Critique. [*Risk Factors for Alcoholism and Alcohol Problems Among Employed Women and Men,* by D.A. Parker & J. A. Brody]. *Occupational Alcoholism: A Review of Research Issues* (p. 132). Rockville, MD: NIAAA.

Rachel, V. (1985). *A women like you: Life stories of women recovering from alcoholism and addiction.* New York: Harper & Row.

Solomon, L. J. (1984). Working women and stress. In C. M. Brody (Ed.). *Women therapists working with women* (pp. 135–144). New York: Springer.

Thoreson, R. W. (1984). The professor at risk: Alcohol/abuse in academe. *Journal of Higher Education, 55*(1), 56–72.

U.S. Department of Health and Human Services. (1987). *Sixth special report to U.S. Congress on alcohol and health.* Rockville, MD: U.S. Government Print Office.

VandenBos, G. R., & Duthie, R. F. (1986). Confronting and supporting colleagues in distress. In R. R. Kilburg, P. E. Nathan, & R. W. Thoreson (Eds.). Professionals in distress: Issues, syndromes and solutions in psychology (pp. 211–231). Washington, D. C.: American Psychological Association.

8

The Use of Group Therapy for Assisting the Recovery and Reentry of Impaired Nurses

Ruth Robinson Staten and Pamela Billings Farley

The problem of impairment in nursing has been well defined in earlier chapters. One question which arises in examining this problem is whether or not there are aspects inherent to the profession of nursing that may contribute to or inhibit recovery from impairment. Although this question has not been satisfactorily answered, work-related issues are usually involved when impaired practice occurs (Naegle, 1984). These issues, as they relate to group psychotherapy, will be explored in this chapter. Group therapy is presented as one modality for promoting the recovery of the impaired nurse both as an individual and as a professional.

Nurses Assisting Nurses, NAN, is a project based in Lexington, Kentucky developed to address the problem of nurse impairment. The project was initiated by a faculty member at the University of Kentucky College of Nursing, who recognized the need for such a project while counseling an impaired nurse. The project has three major foci: education, research, and counseling. The project team consists of nurses prepared at the master's or doctoral level. All are volunteer counselors, employed by a variety of institutions in the area. The project is funded through contributions from nursing organizations, individuals, and a grant from a private foundation. NAN accepted its first client in January, 1984, following 18 months of planning and development. All clients accepted into the project agree to participate in research, as well as to receive counseling services, for which no fee is charged. These services include a 24-hr telephone help line, screening and referral, individual counseling, and group therapy. A major component of the counseling focus is group therapy.

NAN groups consist of six to eight clients and two co-therapists. Group membership is relatively stable with few dropouts or additions. Groups are open-ended. They meet weekly for 1 to 1½ hr. A client's membership in group is not restricted or time limited; some clients have participated in group for up to two years; others have been ready to leave after six months.

An impaired nurse is defined by the project team as a person whose usual level of personal and/or professional functioning has been compromised as a result of substance abuse and/or emotional stress. From the outset of NAN's group therapy sessions, it became readily apparent that certain professional expectations of nurses conflicted with the expectations of the NAN therapy group. To better understand the dynamics of the conflict between these expectations, the norms for certain professional behavior were identified and counternorms for group behavior were offered. Norms are defined as a standard of behavior for group members. There are four norms within nursing that may contribute to impairment or inhibit the recovery process of impaired nurses. These norms are altruism, perfectionism, powerlessness, and denial of feelings.

Counternorms must be offered in group therapy to promote individual and group growth and to enhance the recovery process of clients. Growth, in this situation, is defined as insight into feelings, thoughts, and behaviors with subsequent change toward a healthier lifestyle. Healthier lifestyle includes assertiveness, decrease in stress and stress-related problems, mood elevation, and abstinence from alcohol or other mood-altering substances, as well as exhibiting desired norms. These norms, which are the opposite of the norms of the nursing profession, are acceptance of nurturing, acceptance of strengths and limitations, empowerment, and expression of feelings. Although they may be common to many therapy groups, the norms must be identified, described, and examined within the context of professional nursing. Special effort must be made to reinforce behaviors that enhance both the group psychotherapeutic process and recovery of the individual nurse.

Group Norms

Groups play a powerful role in influencing the behavior and expectations of members. Group norms can have positive or negative effects on members (van Serwellen, 1984). Positive effects are those that meet individual needs while supporting the group goals. Negative effects are those that do not meet the individual needs and may or may not support the group goals. Norms evolve through shared expectations and collaborative efforts of the group, including the therapist. Establishment of norms begins early and, initially, the nurse therapist is in an influential position to determine them. This is especially true when the norms of a smaller group (therapy group) run counter to those of a larger organization (nursing) (Greenberg-Edelstein, 1986). These norms exert pressure on the individual to comply and are held as standards for acceptable behavior. The therapist must recognize not only which norms are desirable but must recognize the effects of all norms on the individual and the group.

The nursing profession can be considered a group whose norms have long been established. The norms for women's conduct as established by our society also contribute to the behavioral expectations that nurses must meet as members of the group of nursing.

Both professional and social norms, then, can have positive or negative effects on nurses. Some of nursing's norms may contribute to the development of impairment within nursing. Some norms may also be counterproductive to the recovery of those nurses who suffer impaired functioning.

Reframing Norms Within Group Sessions

Essential to the process of reframing norms is the establishment and communication of guidelines. These guidelines are discussed with clients at the inception of the group and are repeated as new members join the group. Clients are also given a copy of the guidelines with brief explanations. The following are the major guidelines used in NAN groups:

Take responsibility for your feelings and thoughts.
If you want to talk to an individual, talk to an individual.
If you want to talk to the group, talk to the group.
Stay with your thoughts and feelings in the here and now.
Be aware of your total responses.
Be willing to risk as much honesty as you can.
Be willing to check out your perceptions.
Listening is as important as talking.
Grow in recognizing your patterns of response and behavior.
Don't speak for someone else.
What is said in group stays there.
(Nurses Assisting Nurses, 1984).

During group, the established norms of nursing are identified specifically. The counternorms of acceptance of nurturing, acceptance of strengths and weaknesses, empowerment, and expression of feelings are introduced early and frequently explored. Discussion focuses not only on how the nurse internalizes professional expectations, but includes the effects of these norms on nursing as a group.

Altruism Versus Acceptance of Nurturing

Altruism is a word that might be synonymous with nursing. In fact, a recent media report stated that fewer women are choosing "the altruistic profession of nursing" (Doctors and nurses, 1987). Integrating this characteristic in nursing may affect the development of and recovery from impairment in nursing. Janet Muff (1982) defines altruism as "the philosophy of valuing others higher than one's self" (p. 236). Ruth Greenberg-Edelstein (1986) describes altruism as the most nonreciprocal fundamental level of nurturance. She goes on to explain that this fundamental act of nurturing is based on one's ability to give without the expectation of reciprocity.

This self-sacrificing philosophy is promulgated in many ways in the nursing profession—beginning with basic nursing preparation—and it is reinforced throughout nursing careers (Muff, 1982). "Nurses are the example of altruism par excellence"(Greenberg-Edelstein, 1986). The impaired nurse, too, excels in putting others' needs before her own. Basic demands on nurses reinforce altruism as a desired expectation. Nurses are expected to work overtime, often without compensation. They are asked to work on days off, for extended hours, and during breaks and meals. These are only the more obvious examples of the expectations of altruism. Nurses are taught to put patients' needs and feelings above their own (Muff, 1982). Yet they receive little encouragement or information about expressing their own needs and feelings.

These behaviors and others which are part of the profession's expectations of nurses to be altruistic, are displayed by the impaired nurse, not only in practice, but through participation in group therapy. Many times the impaired nurse is more than willing to take on the role of quasi-group leader, putting others' needs before her own. For many groups, this type of behavior may be desirable and reinforced as members learn to reach outside themselves to others (Greenberg-Edelstein, 1986). For the impaired nurse, it is a natural role—one that has been reinforced throughout professional life—and it may lead to a lack of recognition of the nurse's own needs, which in turn leads to an inability to meet both professional and personal needs.

All too often the impaired nurse is willing to listen and advise someone else—someone whose crisis, feelings, or problems seem greater than her own. Frequently in group therapy, members will try to focus all the time and energy of the group upon the person displaying the most help-seeking behaviors. At the same time, members may be suppressing their own need for nurturance.

Another behavior that stems from altruism is the impaired nurse's inability to seek nurturance from the group. Often the impaired nurse will bring up issues, concerns, or relate crises that occurred weeks earlier. When confronted with why group nurturance was not sought at the time of the event, responses may vary—but all stem from the altruistic nature inherent in the professional role. Examples of altruistic thinking which may interfere with seeking help are "I didn't want to bother anyone" or "everyone has problems of his or her own."

The nurse therapist must be aware of altruistic behaviors and confront the nurse whose behaviors may interfere with seeking and accepting nurturance. Altruistic behaviors must be reframed to help the impaired nurse seek and accept nurturance.

Nurturance includes numerous behaviors. Support, caring, helping, comforting, nursing, and promoting development and growth are frequently associated with nurturance. For those group members who have not experienced adequate nurturing in the past and who do not have the internal support for building nurturing relationships, individual therapy may be necessary for remediation (Greenberg-Edelstein, 1986).

The nurse therapist can establish the counternorm to altruism of acceptance of nurturing by setting the expectation that each member will participate, each member will talk about and for herself and will bring concerns to the group at the time they are occurring. When this behavior does not occur, reasons must be sought. The impaired nurse must be assisted in understanding factors that interfere with seeking and accepting nurturance. Since altruism is so ingrained in the nurse, acceptance of nurturing may be slow, and initial attempts will likely be inconsistent.

Group members are encouraged to help each other identify and explore feelings and events that require nurturing. They are encouraged and helped to use a benevolent and reciprocal approach to provide nurturing to each other. After several attempts at receiving nurturance, the impaired nurse can usually express the positive feelings that come from reciprocal nurturing, such as "this feels good, I like being able to ask for and accept support." The nurse may express feelings of warmth, nurturance, energy, and being cared for.

Case Illustration

In a group of seven members, five attended consistently. The other two members attended only when they were in crisis, extremely emotional, and displaying a high level of help-seeking behavior. Initially, the regular group members would focus all energies and attention on the "distraught member." After several episodes with each of the inconsistent members, the regular members began to discuss their feelings related to changes that would take place when the two inconsistent members attended. Many group sessions were devoted to understanding why the group would allow "one person to take over the group." They began to see that they allowed and encouraged the help-seeking behaviors to dominate the group. Soon the group members were able to connect what happened in group with the altruistic expectations in their work setting and professional roles. Only after the group members could identify and link their behavior and feelings to their professional identity could they discuss how they would like to change their behavior in response to the two members who attended irregularly. They would offer nurturing to the member but would then say, "I have something I need to talk about." They let the members who attended irregularly know that the group could be more helpful if they would attend consistently. From these discussions, members also identified professional expectations that could create uncomfortable feelings.

Perfectionism Versus Acceptance of Strengths and Limitations

In the nursing profession, perfectionism frequently results from a desire to please others. Nurses, the great majority of whom are women, must struggle not only to overcome their reduced status in society vis-à-vis men, but they must also deal with their reduced status vis-à-vis physicians (Bush & Kjervik, 1979; Roberts, 1983). Lack of self-esteem is predominant among nurses. Nurses are expected to be caretakers, nurturers, givers. They are taught and are expected to care for others, accept responsibility, be accountable, yet maintain subservience and passivity (Bush & Kjervik, 1979).

Unrealistic expectations of the nurse begin in the educational process. It is common for the nursing student in the academic setting to make better grades in general courses than in her nursing courses. Nursing is viewed as one of the "tough" major areas of study in college, requiring long study hours and dedication (Meissner, 1986). Future nurses are told they must meet exacting requirements—as part of NURSING. Upon entering the practice setting, nurses are expected to fulfill a variety of roles simultaneously. In one study, eight separate roles expected of nurses in three practice settings were identified: (1) provider of psychological/social support to patient, family, and significant others; (2) teacher of patient, family, or significant others by providing health care instruction or information; (3) coordinator and planner of nursing care; (4) supervisor and administrator of nursing care; (5) documenter of patient care by recording or exchanging information on behalf of the patient; (6) maintainer of professional standards; (7) agent of control, assuring cooperation with nursing and medical care management; and (8) patient advocate (Gorman & Clark, 1986, p. 131).

The pressure for "perfect performance" is great within the nursing profession, too great for many nurses, and has been associated with impairment (Naegle, 1984).

The impaired-nurse group must reframe the norm of perfectionism to acceptance of limitations and strengths. Rather than striving to be all things to all people, group members are encouraged to recognize their own needs. Unrealistic expectations of self are confronted, and individuals are encouraged to set achievable goals. Initially, it is the task of the nurse therapist to help clients identify unrealistic expectations and to direct the group discussion toward achievable goals for the individual as well as for the group. As members become more insightful and adept at group interaction, they begin to confront and direct each other, needing only support and occasional direction from the nurse therapist.

Case Illustration

For several group sessions, Susan had been quiet, saying she was working a lot of overtime and was just tired. One evening, another group member expressed concern for her and inquired how long Susan was expecting to continue working at this pace. Susan responded that she was reluctant to refuse to work overtime, she felt she "owed" the hospital for hiring her as a recovering nurse and that they expected more of her because of the "favor" they had done for her. She also felt a need to maintain the "super nurse" image because people were watching her performance more closely than that of nonimpaired nurses. Another group member shared her own experience with being "super nurse"—relapse. The group asked Susan if her work schedule was interfering with her recovery program. Susan admitted that she had not been attending her 12-step meetings regularly or talking regularly with her Alcoholics Anonymous sponsor. Susan was then asked which she viewed as more important—"super nurse" or recovery? From this interaction, Susan realized a need to care for herself and asked the group for suggestions about how to approach her supervisor regarding her work schedule. Susan was able to reorganize her time in order to meet her needs while at the same time perform her job competently and fulfill her family responsibilities adequately.

All too frequently nurses who have been striving for perfection have difficulty identifying their strengths. They have failed at being perfect; therefore, they see themselves as failures. Through encouragement, support, and confrontation, members begin to view their strengths and build upon these, rather than focus on limitations.

Case Illustration

During the group meeting, Joan, whose nursing license had recently been reinstated, was discussing her fear of applying for a job in nursing. Her comments included: "Why would they hire me when they could get someone who's not an addict? Then they wouldn't have to bother with urine drug screens or reports to the Board (of nursing). Everybody will talk about me (drug-abuse history)." The group responded to her remarks with questions: "What do you have to offer? What have you gained from your experience with addiction and your recovery process?" They gave information on how they approached their own reentry interviews: "Be honest, matter of fact, and emphasize recovery." Finally, they helped Joan role play an interview, responding with their own ideas and suggestions.

Powerlessness Versus Empowerment

The term "power" is associated with control, influence, and strength (Kelly, 1985, p. 354) and has a negative connotation to some. The term "empower," on the other hand, is defined as "to give faculties or abilities to" (Webster, 1976, p. 744). Nursing is frequently viewed as a powerless, or unempowered, profession. "The majority of practicing nurses are women who have been socialized in female and nursing roles characterized by dependence, passivity, and deference to others in the health care system, particularly to physicians" (American Nurses Association, 1984, p. 5). Women are traditionally viewed as more dependent, vulnerable, nurturing, and supportive than men. The health care system has been characterized as a paternalistic organization in which nurses play the traditional female role (LaMonica, 1983). Much has been written about the "Nurse/Physician Game" in which the nurse must make suggestions about patient care in a passive, nonassertive manner in order to preserve the physician's ego (Bush & Kjervik, 1979; Roberts, 1983). Such a game perpetuates sex role stereotyping by enabling the physician to make decisions and highlighting the passive subservience of nurses. This combination of factors as well as lack of awareness of professional rights is seen as a contribution to nurse impairment (American Nurses Association, 1984).

The nurse therapist must first help impaired-nurse group members to recognize and confront powerless thinking. Behaviors frequently encountered include inadequate preparation for disciplinary procedures—"The Board (of nursing) will act and I'll just have to accept it"—acceptance of poor work environment—"I can't do anything about it (staffing, policy, etc.)"—and acceptance of dysfunctional relationships—"Maybe things will get better or I'll adjust."

In order to reframe the norm of powerlessness, those powers inherent in the individual and the profession must be identified. As members bring issues to the group, the nurse therapist assists the group in identifying choices and then in exploring potential outcomes. When the individual has decided which alternative to implement, the group can then assist in anticipatory guidance through discussion and role playing.

Case Illustration

Ann, a group member, discussed her anger and frustration with a co-worker who was sleeping on the job (night shift). Since Ann was a recovering nurse, recently reentering nursing, she expressed a desire to avoid conflicts, and thus had done nothing about the situation. Beverly, another group member, told Ann that she (Ann) had a responsibility as a professional to address the issue. Susan added that Ann not only had a responsibility, she had a right to expect her co-worker to remain alert and able to assume her share of work and responsibility. The group then helped Ann explore her options and the probable results. Even when Ann decided which alternative she wanted to implement, she still felt uncomfortable. Group members suggested she practice what she wanted to say, then gave her suggestions and encouragement. The following week Ann reported to the group that she had followed through with her plan. The co-worker had made excuses but did not become angry. Her behavior had improved and although she seemed somewhat distant to Ann, they were working together effectively. Ann shared her feelings of relief and pride in herself for being able to confront the situation.

Group members gain a sense of empowerment not only through their own experience, but from other members as well. They, in effect, model empowerment for each other. They share accomplishments, with emphasis on the effect the accomplishment has upon their feelings and self-concept.

Case Illustration

One evening a group member shared the experience of completing her final hearing at the Board of Nursing. The nurse had complied with one year's licensure suspension, followed by two years of probation. At the final hearing, she successfully applied to have her license reinstated without restriction. A fellow group member had her license revoked five years previously and had not applied for reinstatement. She shared her reluctance to ask for reinstatement, fearing failure and rejection. She was encouraged that other group members had regained their licenses and were successfully reentering the profession. This nurse believed that she was now ready to apply for reinstatement and asked for group support during the process.

Denial of Feelings Versus Expression of Feelings

Denial of feelings is closely linked to altruism, perfectionism, and powerlessness. The self-sacrificing nature of nursing is just one of the contributing factors in the development of denial of feelings (Estes & Heinemann, 1986). Beginning with basic educational preparation and continuing into professional careers, nurses are taught that close control over emotions is essential to being a "good" nurse. The quest for perfection keeps the nurse constantly aware of the expectation that emotions must not interfere with the ability to give high-quality patient care. Technical expertise and ideas are more highly valued than feelings (Skevington, 1984). Those emotions that are expressed receive little if any attention because of the nurse's powerless position within the health care hierarchy and society at large.

Most nurses can recall the moment when they were told that expression of feelings was not acceptable. Many times when a nurse is experiencing a strong emotional response she "may conclude that there is something wrong with herself rather than with the situation in which she finds herself" (Skevington, 1984, p. 53). This expectation leads the nurse to suppress those feelings deemed unacceptable. Such feelings may include anger, guilt, resentment, boredom, remorse, loneliness, and anxiety (Estes & Heinemann, 1986, p. 293).

NAN group members often relate events that have occurred or thoughts they have had since the last session. Frequently, these are highly emotional situations, such as the death of a patient or confrontation with a colleague. The group member often presents the situation in an intellectual, emotionless manner.

The impaired nurse may respond to questioning about her lack of emotional response with statements as "How I feel about it is nothing compared with how the patient and the family are feeling" (altruism). The group member may say that such situations are just part of the job and must be accepted (powerlessness). The impaired nurse also tends to negate any feelings she has by stating "everyone else can handle it so why shouldn't I?" (perfectionism).

Denial of feelings is compounded by the tendency of substance abusers and those around them to deny problems, thus preventing help seeking (Estes & Heinemann, 1986; Naegle, 1984). Corrective emotional experiences (expression of feelings) are an essential factor in the curative process for all those who seek group psychotherapy (Yalom, 1975).

Denial of feelings may be the most deep-seated, complex norm that the nurse therapist must reframe. This difficult task is not an unusual one for group therapists in general, however. A wide range of expectations may be employed to create the norm of expression of feelings. The most essential aspect in assisting the impaired nurse to begin expressing suppressed emotions is to provide an atmosphere of trust and unconditional acceptance (Estes & Heinemann, 1986; Greenberg-Edelstein, 1986; Skevington, 1984; van Serwellen, 1984; Yalom, 1975). These expectations can be stated in the guidelines and reaffirmed by the nurse therapist with role modeling behaviors. Risk taking of this nature is especially critical at this point since the impaired nurse tends to believe that any expression of unstable negative emotions may be interpreted as relapse. As the group develops, its members will help each other by pointing out specific behaviors in each other that they have come to recognize as behavioral expressions of certain emotions.

Case Illustration

> One group became so in-tune with each other they could tell when one member was struggling emotionally by the way in which she carried her purse into group. When group members pointed this occurrence out to their peer, she was initially defensive, and denied difficulties. Over time, and with much persistence by other members, she was able to express her feelings to the group.

Group members assist each other in recognizing, identifying, and verbally expressing a wide range of emotions. The impaired nurse will express a sense of relief when she is finally able to release emotions in a safe and supportive environment. The group, with the assistance of the nurse therapist, must explore how this norm is reinforced in the work setting and the effects it has within the profession.

Transference of Counternorms Outside the Group

As has been noted, there is obvious overlapping of norms, counternorms, and their associated issues. The norms of perfectionism and altruism are perhaps the most closely aligned of the four, and in fact are frequently displayed together, for it is in the altruistic behaviors that nurses strive to be most perfect. As the impaired nurse begins to embrace norms counter to the familiar and valued ones previously held, the nurse therapist must be available to guide and assist, for displaying counternorms outside NAN group frequently creates anxiety. Maintaining individual values in face of pressure to conform is difficult.

Expression of feelings is often the first counternorm to be evidenced. As the impaired nurse becomes more adept at identifying and expressing feelings within the group setting, she begins to explore the option of doing so in other settings. This is generally better accepted in personal situations than in work situations. Other health care professionals may be uncomfortable when a nurse exhibits behaviors (expressing feelings) counter to the expected norm. In role modeling expression of feelings appropriately, the impaired nurse can affect the norms of the profession.

Letting go of altruism is very difficult for group members, and it is in fact desirable to retain some altruistic behaviors. With time and effort, however, group members have been able to set limits upon meeting the needs of others to the exclusion of their own. The ability to recognize one's own needs and set about meeting them grows with time. In the majority of cases, this has created less stress in professional situations than in personal ones. Family members may have difficulty adjusting to the new behaviors, but most do realize the long-term benefit.

Perfectionism is also a most difficult norm for the impaired nurse to reframe. Those nurses reentering practice especially feel internal, as well as external, pressure for excellence. The recovering nurse who becomes more confident and comfortable in the workplace can begin to relax and perform at an acceptable (but imperfect) level.

With every success the nurse has with empowerment, the more comfortable she becomes. Even when efforts are not successful, the experience of taking action rather than being passive leads to improved self-esteem and increased comfort with assertive behaviors. Empowerment creates only minimal conflict in either personal or professional situations for those nurses who embrace it.

Implications for the Nurse Therapist

Although having nurses serve as group therapists is essential to the exploration and understanding of norms and their effects on impairment and the profession, it also creates some challenges. The nurse therapist as a member of the nursing profession has likely adopted or adapted to the norms of altruism, perfectionism, powerlessness, and denial of feelings. The nurse therapist must be constantly aware of her own behaviors and work toward integrating the desirable counter norms of acceptance of nurturing, acceptance of strengths and weaknesses, empowerment, and expression of feelings within this group. The nurse therapist must recognize and help group members build upon the positive aspects inherent to our profession. The primary function is to assist the impaired nurse to meet client or patient needs in conjunction with meeting her own. To do so, the nurse therapist uses the impaired nurse therapy group to reframe norms of the profession which may contribute to impairment, or inhibit recovery. Counternorms must be established to promote individual growth, growth of the nurse therapist, group growth, and, ideally, growth of the profession of nursing.

References

Bush, M. A., & Kjervik, D. K. (1979). The nurse's self image. In D. K. Kjervik & I. M. Martinson (Eds.), *Women in stress: A nursing perspective* (pp. 46–58). Norwalk, CT: Appleton-Century-Crofts.

Doctors and nurses. *Herald Leader.*(1987, March 20). Lexington, KY.

Estes, N., & Heinemann, E. (1986). *Alcoholism: Development, consequences, and intervention.* St. Louis: C.V. Mosby.

Gorman, S. A., & Clark, N. M. (1986). Power and effective nursing practice. *Nursing Outlook, 34*(3), 129–134.

Greenberg-Edelstein, R. (1986). *The nurturance phenomenon—the roots of group psychotherapy.* Norwalk, CT: Appleton-Century-Crofts.

Kelly, L. Y. (1985). *Dimensions of professional nursing.* New York: McMillan.

LaMonica, E. L. (1983). The nurse as helper: Today and tomorrow. In N. L. Chaska (Ed.), *The nursing profession: A time to speak* (pp. 489–499). New York: McGraw Hill.

Meissner, J. E. (1986). Nurses are we eating our young? *Nursing 86, 16*(3), 51–53.

Muff, J. (1982). *Socialization, sexism and stereotyping—women's issues in nursing.* St. Louis: C. V. Mosby Co.

Naegle, M. (Ed.). (1984). *Addictions and psychological dysfunctions in nursing. The profession's response to the problem.* Kansas City, MO: American Nurses Association.

Roberts, S. J. (1983). Oppressed group behavior: Implications for nursing. *Advances in Nursing Science, 5*(4), 21–30.

Skevington, S. (1984). *Understanding nurses.* New York: Wiley.

van Servellen, G. (1984). *Group and family therapy.* St. Louis: C. V. Mosby.

Webster's third new international dictionary. (1976). Springfield, MA: G. & C. Merriam Co.

Wilson, R. (Ed.). (1983). *Group guidelines.* Unpublished Guidelines for NAN Project. Lexington, KY: Nurses Assisting Nurses.

Yalom, I. (1975). *The theory and practice of group psychotherapy* (3rd ed.). New York: Basic Books.

9

Self-Help Groups for Nurses

Patricia L. Green

Dependence on alcohol or other drugs is a chronic, potentially fatal illness that is subject to relapse. For that reason a method of ongoing support for sobriety assures the greatest potential for recovery. Even the best treatment program can only assist in the beginning of the recovery process. Whether this process continues will depend upon the support the nurse receives following formal treatment. In his text, *The Natural History of Alcoholism* (1983), George Vaillant quotes the work of J. D. Frank, *Persuasion and Healing: A Comparative Study of Psychotherapy,* "If attitude change is to be maintained, repetition of group rituals and the group support that they engender must be sustained after clinic discharge."

For nurses in the early stage of chemical dependency, particularly for alcoholics, attendance at a support group such as Alcoholics Anonymous (AA) or Narcotics Anonymous (NA) may be all the treatment that is needed. For other nurses who may be in need of professional inpatient treatment, but lack the ability to pay for it, an AA or NA group or a support group for nurses may be all that is accessible.

This chapter discusses the various support groups available for nurses and how they may be of benefit. The differences between the groups will be outlined, and information about how to make a referral to one of them will be provided.

Why Support Groups Are Important

The negative attitude of some members of the nursing profession toward alcoholics and drug addicts has been discussed in the literature (Ferneau & Morton, 1968) and earlier in this book. By "negative attitude" it is meant that alcoholics and drug addicts are viewed as being weak-willed and immoral. The image of the drunken nurse portrayed by Charles Dickens' character, "Sairy Gamp," is still held by vast numbers of nurses. Nursing education has not provided information about addictive disease as a primary process in and of itself (Bissell & Haberman, 1984; Burkhalter, 1975; Einstein & Wolfson, 1970). Rather, nurses have been educated in regard to the physical consequences of excessive use of alcohol or other drugs; the etiology of the illness has been variously explained as stemming from lack of will power or psychiatric illness. Alcoholics and drug addicts have been traditionally viewed as "premorbidly passive, dependent, latently homosexual, sociopathic, 'oral-dependent,' and fearful of intimacy" (Vaillant, 1983). Treatment has been directed toward admonishments to "cut down" or "control" use, or toward the solution of the perceived underlying problems. Given this belief system within the profession, it is small wonder that "alcoholism or drug addiction" is an accusation rather than a diagnosis, and nurses are reluctant to accept the reality of their own addiction.

Because of these negative attitudes, few nurses in recovery are willing to have their recovering status known, and many (if not most) nurses entering a treatment program have never known a recovering alcoholic or drug addict, much less a recovering nurse. Identifying oneself as an alcoholic or addict is an important first step in recovery. This process is facilitated if the person is placed in association with other persons who have begun a recovery and are willing to talk openly about their experience. This association helps replace the negative image of the alcoholic or drug addict as a skid-row bum with a positive one of a recovering person leading a productive, functional life. These groups supply the essential ingredients of acceptance and hope (Blume cited in Zimberg, Wallace, & Blume, 1978).

Isolation is an important factor associated with addictive disease. As the disease progresses, the alcoholic or addict becomes more and more estranged from other persons, in part as the result of the negative behaviors that occur, but also to conceal the extent of the drinking or drug use. This isolation serves to reinforce and perpetuate the drinking or drug use. An ongoing support group is a valuable method of ending the isolation, helping to integrate the person back into social relationships (Blume cited in Zimberg, Wallace, & Blume, 1978).

There is no research to support the belief that the guilt experienced by nurses who become addicted to alcohol or other drugs is greater than that of other alcoholics or drug addicts. However, in this author's experience, many persons who work with addicted nurses believe that it is and view this guilt as a treatment issue with the nurse. Nursing has its origins in religious orders and the military, both of which emphasize self-discipline and self-sacrifice. Considering that most nurses have been taught little about the addictive disease process, it is not difficult to believe that guilt is an important factor to be considered in efforts to help the nurse. Association with other persons (and most particularly other nurses) who have had the same experience helps the addicted nurse facilitate the process of self-forgiveness.

The psychological defense mechanisms found in addictive disease such as impaired perception of reality, denial, rationalization, intellectualization, and withdrawal can be confronted very effectively in a group setting. Indeed, many persons working in the field of chemical dependency treatment consider group therapy the treatment of choice. The group members learn from each other and develop self-awareness and problem-solving ability. For most of the support groups, this assistance is available at no financial cost. Furthermore, it is this author's opinion that even the best individual psychotherapy cannot provide the depth and richness of experience afforded by regular attendance at a group with other recovering persons.

In addition to the general benefits of participating in a 12-step group such as AA or NA (described later in this chapter) that are important for all addicted persons, it is helpful for nurses also to attend a group limited to nurses. Nurses tend to be reluctant to talk about the issues related to nursing in a group of nonnurses. As discussed above, nurses are frequently ashamed of being addicted to alcohol or other drugs, and they will protect the image of nursing to the detriment of their own recovery. In the setting of a group of other recovering nurses, they may feel free to discuss their feelings about their addiction and also the issues that are frequently present with regard to the potential or actual loss of licensure. Other alcoholics or drug addicts may lose a job but seldom their profession, as does the health professional whose license to practice may be suspended or revoked.

Another issue unique to recovering nurses (and recovering physicians as well) is that of the real or potential harm done to patients while the nurse's practice is impaired by alcohol or other drugs. In addition to the guilt of being an addicted nurse, the recovering nurse must face this most difficult admission. The denial of harm to patients is very strong, and many recovering nurses continue to cling to it far into their recovery process. Certainly, most nurses will not want to admit or discuss it in an AA or NA meeting with nonnurses present. A support group of other recovering nurses is the optimal setting for catharsis and healing. This process should be facilitated, but the nurse should not be confronted heavily with these issues early in recovery when a forced exploration of painful issues may precipitate a return to the use of the chemical (Brown, 1985).

There are several different types of groups available to nurses for support of recovery. The most widely available is AA or its counterpart for drug addicts. There are also therapy groups, some specifically for nurses. In the past few years there has been a proliferation of support groups for nurses that do not fall within the framework of either AA/NA or group psychotherapy.

Therapy Groups for Nurses

Therapy groups may be operated by a treatment center and facilitated by a professional on a fee-for-service basis, or the group may be provided as the aftercare component of a total treatment package. Many chemical dependency treatment centers are now advertising treatment programs especially for nurses. The program offered is generally the generic treatment program provided to all their patients with a focus on the treatment issues that pertain to nurses. These issues are addressed in a group setting with other nurses. Professional therapy groups may also be facilitated by an individual therapist in private practice, although there are few of these at the present time (National Nurses Society on Addictions, 1987).

Nonprofessional Support Groups

At the present time, at least 30 states have support groups for nurses (National Nurses Society on Addictions, 1987). A few are considered to provide professional therapy but the vast majority do not. Support groups that consider themselves as providing support rather than therapy often operate under the auspices of a chemical-dependency treatment center or a peer-assistance program. In states lacking formal assistance programs for nurses, the groups may be facilitated by recovering nurses operating independently in an effort to assist other nurses into recovery and to monitor that recovery for employers. These groups have frequently become the nucleus for the development of a formal peer assistance or diversion program for nurses in the state.

The format of support groups will vary depending on the sponsoring agency. Some may be considered therapy as outlined above, others may be AA or NA groups with membership limited to nurses. Most of the support groups that are based on neither therapy nor AA/NA list their goals and expectations for the group, and members agree to these when they begin attending. This is more formal than AA or NA where persons attend without making any formal commitment.

One reason for the increased number of nurse support groups is the rather unique nature of their members' addiction. While many of the nurses have used narcotics parenterally, they do not identify with the "street-wise" drug addicts who attend Narcotics Anonymous meetings. These nurses' style of life may be more similar to that of the members of Alcoholics Anonymous who are traditionally uncomfortable with "hard" drug addicts. Members of AA cling to the

Twelve Traditions of AA, which state that the primary purpose of the group is to "carry its message to the *alcoholic* who still suffers" (Alcoholics Anonymous, 1976). Persons in early recovery are very sensitive to rejection, and although some AA groups are tolerant of drug addicts in their meetings, others are not. Persons referring nurses to these groups should be well informed of the orientation of the groups in their area. Another factor to be considered is that patterns of drug use considered "acceptable" to society have changed. The use of cocaine by the middle and upper classes, as well as the widespread use of minor tranquilizers that may lead to addiction is blurring the traditional distinction between drug addicts and alcoholics. Many alcoholics beginning recovery today have used drugs as well as alcohol.

Many of the therapy or independent support groups (but not AA or NA) monitor nurses' recovery for employers or state boards of nursing. There is some question whether this is appropriate, since much of the benefit of a group is having a "safe" setting in which one is free to self-disclose and where confidentiality is assured. If a nurse knows that a relapse into drinking or drug use will be reported, the group process, in which honesty is a necessity, will be inhibited. On the other hand, it is the experience of persons facilitating these groups that attendance at the group is erratic unless attendance is required. A solution to this dilemma is to separate the monitoring function from the support function. The person who monitors the nurse's compliance with the terms and conditions of the agreement does so outside the group setting. The group facilitator reports to the state board of nursing or the employer only whether or not the nurse is attending, not the content of the nurse's activity in the group. The monitor could be the Employee Assistance Counselor at the workplace, a representative of a formal Peer Assistance Program, or a staff member of the State Board of Nursing.

Persons contemplating the implementation of a support group that will operate outside the structure of AA or NA should plan to address these issues. Goals and objectives of the group should be clear from the beginning. The nurse must be told who will be informed in regard to attendance or relapse. It should also be remembered that nurses coming into these groups in early recovery are apt to be angry and manipulative, especially if they are being required to attend, and group facilitator(s) need support and guidance as well.

A treatment issue that sometimes arises with nurses (and other health professionals) is their belief that they are in some respect different from other alcoholics and drug addicts. This may be a vestige of denial and should be confronted when it occurs. The circumstances of a nurse's life and livelihood may be different, as outlined above, but the disease process is the same as it is for any alcoholic or drug addict. Therefore, it is important that nurses who attend the special support groups for nurses be required to attend a 12-step group (discussed below) in addition to other group participation.

Nontherapy support groups can be very helpful for the reasons outlined above, but it should be remembered that they are not treatment and should be employed as an adjunct to professional treatment and regular attendance at AA or NA.

Self-Help Groups

In 1935 a physician and a stock broker agreed to help each other maintain sobriety; from that meeting Alcoholics Anonymous was born. From this beginning the so-called "self-help" group was formed. Its use has spread so that now its principles are used to treat many other illnesses or compulsive disorders such as over-eating, gambling, child abuse, sexual dysfunction, and emotional illness. The term "so-called" self-help is employed because members of these groups object to its use to describe them. One of the tenets of a 12-step group such as AA is that it is only when the addicted person stops trying to get well by reliance solely on self or "will power" and becomes willing to turn to others for help that recovery begins (Alcoholics Anonymous, 1976). Because AA was the first of these groups and is by far the largest in terms of membership, and also because it was the model after which the other groups were patterned, it will be used as the prototype to explain how the 12-step groups work. Similarities and differences with the other groups will be discussed later in the chapter.

Alcoholics Anonymous

Many helping professionals are supportive of AA but do not understand how it works and view it as "folk therapy." In her research study of alcoholism in 407 physicians, nurses, social workers, dentists, and college women, Bissell found that only 11% of the medical professionals, one social worker, and no attorneys had learned anything about AA in their professional training (Bissell & Haberman, 1984). Further, she found that they held stereotypical views of alcoholics in AA as "skid row" types or religious fanatics. Many believed AA was a group of people who substituted dependence on alcohol with an equally unhealthy dependence on AA.

Similarities and Differences Between AA and Group Therapy

Brown (1985) also discusses the lack of understanding of AA by psychotherapists and outlines the similarities and differences between AA and therapy. She emphasizes the benefits to be gained when both are used in the treatment of the alcoholic, and states that the goal of both is personal autonomy. "What happens in AA is what happens in good psychotherapy: increased self-knowledge and the potential for change. The function and the process of change are similar, although the forms and language may differ" (pp. 267–280).

AA meetings are highly ritualized whereas group therapy is not. Since the AA group operates entirely autonomously and without formal commitment or expectations, this ritual provides the framework within which the group functions. The focus in AA is on cessation of drinking. All of the work that is done through the use of the "steps" of the program is an effort to eliminate the thinking and behavior that may lead back to the use of alcohol as a way to cope.

AA provides a great deal of nurturing and encourages dependency on the group, the steps, a Higher Power, and the sponsor. (The concept of Higher Power and sponsorship is explained later in this section.) It discourages confrontation and interpersonal feedback within the group setting. Older members speak from their own experience and the newly recovering person is free to accept that information and use it or not. In AA, confrontation of maladaptive behavior is done individually by the sponsor. The AA group emphasizes similarities and admonishes the new comer to "identify; don't compare." Members develop self-awareness by observing their own behavior or personality characteristics in other members of the group.

Group therapy, on the other hand, discourages dependency and uses the anxiety that this engenders to facilitate self-awareness. Group members are encouraged to provide direct feedback to each other in interpersonal interaction. Dependency is focused on the group leader through the process of transference, whereas the AA member will meet dependency needs through many different persons.

Basic Assumptions of AA

In order to understand and utilize AA, certain basic assumptions must be outlined. The first and most important is that chemical dependency is a disease, and the only appropriate goal of treatment is total abstinence from all mind-altering drugs. Members of AA believe that alcoholics cannot safely use tranquilizers or smoke marijuana, and drug addicts should not attempt to drink socially. Persons in recovery from chemical dependency believe, based on their experience and that of others in the program, that this will lead to a return to the "drug of choice" or to cross-addiction to another drug. This is a very important issue for recovering nurses who will be expected to produce drug-free body fluids for monitoring purposes. Assertions that alcoholics can return to controlled drinking can be found in the literature (e.g., Armor, Polich, & Stanbul, 1978). However, Bissell's study of alcoholic professionals found that physicians who believed or were undecided about whether an alcoholic can ever return safely to normal drinking relapsed more frequently than those who did not hold this belief (Bissell & Haberman, 1984). Members of AA hold that the continuing belief in the ability to control drinking inhibits the surrender that is a prerequisite to recovery.

Another basic tenant of AA is the belief that there is a spiritual aspect to recovery from alcoholism. This may be interpreted as religious fanaticism by persons who have only a superficial understanding of the AA program. Very simply defined, the spiritual aspect concerns the search for purpose and meaning in life. It is not religious in that there is no dogma or particular set of beliefs that the AA member is required to espouse. The AA program is compatible with organized religion. On the other hand, a number of AA members interpret the idea of a "Higher Power" in humanistic terms, expressed as the belief in something of value larger than themselves (Mack, 1981). One cannot utilize the 12 steps of the AA program unless there is a "surrender" of self-will to some Higher Power, whether that is viewed as a belief in God in the traditional sense or simply as reliance on the AA group and the "program."

The Twelve Steps

Within the scientific community there continues to be controversy about whether or not the personality profile and defense mechanisms the alcoholic presents at the time of treatment were present before the development of the alcoholism (Valliant, 1983). However, it is observed that there is a "preferred defense structure" as Wallace refers to it in the text edited by Zimberg, Wallace, and Blume (1978). AA calls this the "alcoholic personality," and the 12 steps of the program are designed to help the alcoholic become aware of this characteristic behavior and to change it.

Much of the time in AA meetings is spent in discussion of the steps. Working the steps is suggested, not mandatory. (In point of fact none of AA is mandatory, which makes it more palatable to persons who frequently have problems with authority and rebel automatically when told they have to do something.) The steps are written in the past tense, having been developed by the early members of AA and written down after they were found to be effective.

1. We admitted we were powerless over alcohol — that our lives had become unmanageable.
2. We came to believe that a Power Greater than Ourselves could restore us to sanity.
3. We made a decision to turn our will and our lives over to the care of God AS WE UNDERSTOOD HIM.
4. We made a searching and fearless moral inventory of ourselves.
5. We admitted to God, to ourselves and to another human being the exact nature of our wrongs.

6. We were entirely ready to have God remove all these defects of character.
7. We humbly asked Him to remove our shortcomings.
8. We made a list of all persons we had harmed and became willing to make amends to them all.
9. We made direct amends to such persons wherever possible, except when to do so would harm them or others.
10. We continued to take personal inventory and when we were wrong promptly admitted it.
11. We sought through prayer and meditation to improve our conscious contact with God as we understood Him, praying only for knowledge of His will for us and the power to carry it out.
12. Having had a spiritual awakening as a result of these steps, we tried to carry this message to alcoholics and to practice these principles in all our affairs.

Working the steps provides a framework for recovery in which addicted persons admit the reality of the addiction. They recognize the problems and the destruction that has occurred in their lives as a result of drinking or drug use and the behaviors attendant on that use. The person recognizes that outside help is necessary in order to get well. This is an admission that will power alone will be insufficient; that help from a "Higher Power" is necessary. Further, the person decides to get well, which means accepting changes in both attitude and behavior. Embarking on change necessitates that the person take stock of existing personality characteristics, both positive and negative, and make a commitment to work for improvement. Accepting that other persons have been injured as a result of their behavior, recovering persons make apologies or restitution to others as necessary. A commitment to continue to examine their own behavior and to strive for improvement is made, again emphasizing the need for help in doing so. And last comes the recognition of the profound change that has occurred, and they agree to try to help other alcoholics.

The steps are difficult for members to understand in the beginning. As the person struggles with the changes needed and "works" the steps, that understanding will grow and change with time.

Sponsorship

An outgrowth of the twelfth step is the concept of sponsorship. This is a unique arrangement whereby a person who has been in the program for some period of time is asked by a new member to act as a guide in working the program. The sponsor agrees to be available to the sponsoree when needed; the person being sponsored agrees to "work the program." Styles of sponsorship vary, with some sponsors being very strict and confrontive, others more lenient. Newcomers are free to choose sponsors who fit their needs.

Types of Meetings

Types of meetings vary. Some meetings are "closed," meaning only persons who have a desire to stop drinking are welcome; others are "open," meaning anyone may attend. Closed meetings are usually smaller, discussion-type meetings focused on one of the steps or any topic or problem with which a member may be struggling. Open meetings frequently are larger with a member or members giving their "drunkelogue." This is a recounting of the person's life before and during the period of active drinking, what happened to precipitate the beginning of recovery, and what life is like now that the person is working the program.

Anonymity

Since alcoholism was severely stigmatized when the group began (1935), the assurance of anonymity was a prerequisite for AA's growth and survival. Although there has been progress in the recognition that alcoholism is an illness, the stigma still remains, making openness about recovery difficult. As shown earlier, nursing continues to stigmatize the alcoholic or drug addict, and chemically dependent nurses frequently guard their anonymity closely. Members use only their first name and initial of the last and are never pressured to reveal more about themselves than they are willing to share.

Traditions

AA is very loosely constructed. The organization is guided by the Twelve Traditions of the program, as the lives of the individual members are guided by the Twelve Steps. The Traditions state the following principles: The primary purpose is to carry the message to the still-suffering alcoholic. AA does not affiliate with other groups or lend its name to causes. It remains autonomous and will not accept contributions from outside sources. The focus is on achieving and maintaining sobriety through individuals "working the program," which means attending meetings, working the steps, and reaching out to other alcoholics (Alcoholics Anonymous, 1953).

Other 12-Step Groups

As mentioned above, the model of AA as a program of recovery has been adopted by persons suffering from other illnesses or compulsive disorders. Narcotics Anonymous was the first of these and has been joined by Overeaters Anonymous, Gamblers Anonymous, Cocaine Anonymous, Emotions Anonymous, and Parents Anonymous for abusive parents. There are also several groups for anorexia nervosa and bulimia. These groups follow the outline for structure and program described above for AA.

Alanon

AA has emphasized the importance of the family from the beginning of the program. The earliest members of AA were male; their wives met with them in the beginning but very early on found that their needs were better served when they met separately. Thus, Alanon was organized separately and distinctly from AA but parallel to it. Alanon is available to anyone who has some relationship to an alcoholic (or Naranon for families of drug addicts). This person is usually a spouse, parent, or child but may also include friend or employer. Members of Alanon work the same steps as the alcoholics, focusing on their own behavior rather than that of the alcoholic and recognizing the futility of trying to control the alcoholic or the alcoholic's drinking.

It is being recognized that living with an active alcoholic can result in impairment for the nurse who is married to an alcoholic. Vaillant makes the statement, "Outside of residence in a concentration camp, there are very few sustained human experiences that make one the recipient of as much sadism as does being a close family member of an alcoholic" (Valliant, 1983, p. 20). It is not difficult to understand that the practice of a nurse living in such a situation may be adversely affected. I have heard of cases in which a nurse diverted drugs from the workplace to take home to an addicted relative. Some peer assistance programs for nurses now include these nurses in their program.

Women for Sobriety

In 1975 a group for female alcoholics, Women for Sobriety (WFS), was established. It was founded by a psychologist, Jean Kirkpatrick, who wrote of her recovery in a book, *Turnabout: Help for a New Life* (Kirkpatrick, 1986). Kirkpatrick believes that AA was designed for the male alcoholic and does not meet the needs of women alcoholics. WFS has its own set of "Thirteen Statements" rather than steps. The focus is on self-affirmation and the achievement of self-esteem. Groups are found in various part of the country and can be located using the address listed in the Appendix of Self-Help Groups in this chapter.

Referral to Support Groups

When an attempt is made to refer someone to any of the support groups described above, it is essential that the referring person be knowledgeable about the group, the auspices under which it functions, and how it works. It is also imperative that the referring person believe that the group can help the nurse to recover. If the person referring has doubts about the efficacy of the program or disagrees with its philosophy, these feelings are likely to be communicated to the chemically dependent nurse. Attending a new group for the first time is very-anxiety arousing. Any indication that the group may not work for them is likely to be seized upon as an excuse not to attend, or to discount its efficacy before a fair trial. For readers not familiar with AA or NA, it is suggested that meetings open to the public be attended. A recovering member of an AA or NA group could be sought out and used as a resource in "12-stepping" newly recovering nurses. The most positive advocate for any program is someone who has been helped by it. If that someone is a recovering nurse, so much the better.

Newly recovering nurses may also be reluctant to attend one of the support groups limited to nurses. This is in part a fear of the censure of other nurses, but also because it is frightening to hear about the experiences of nurses who have had their licenses suspended or revoked. Attending these groups makes it difficult to maintain a denial system. When a nurse is still in heavy denial there will be resistance to association with persons who are not. Referring persons must be aware of this dynamic. If the nurse is not required to attend (by a peer-assistance program or state board of nursing or as part of a return to work contract with an employer), it may be helpful to negotiate a trial contract for a period of 90 days. Frequently by the end of this period, the nurse will appreciate the value of the group and will continue to attend. Contracting to attend for 90 days will seem more acceptable in the beginning than being "sentenced" for life.

Contact with groups may be made in a variety of ways. AA or NA groups may be located by consulting the telephone directory. Cities and towns of any size have AA groups and more and more now have NA groups. In addition, treatment centers may be able to help with information. Cities that have a local chapter of the National Council of Alcoholism can supply information about groups as well as treatment centers. Specialty support groups such as Women for Sobriety, Overeaters Anonymous, and other are listed in the Appendix of Self-Help Groups in this chapter.

To locate support groups especially for nurses, it is suggested that readers contact their State Nurses Association. In addition, the Impaired Nurse Committee of the National Nurses Society on Addictions maintains a national network of resources. These resources may be obtained by contacting the number also listed in the Appendix of Self-Help Groups.

References

Alcoholics Anonymous. (1953). *Twelve steps and twelve traditions.* New York: Alcoholics Anonymous World Services, Inc.

Alcoholics Anonymous. (1957). *Alcoholics Anonymous Comes of Age: A Brief History of AA*. New York: Alcoholics Anonymous World Services, Inc.

Alcoholics Anonymous. (1976). *Alcoholics Anonymous* (3rd ed.). New York: Alcoholics Anonymous World Services, Inc.

Armour, D. J., Polich, J. M., & Stanbul, H. B. (1978). *Alcoholism and Treatment*. New York: Wiley.

Bissell, L., & Haberman, P. (1984). *Alcoholism in the Professions.* New York: Oxford University Press.

Brown, S. (1985). *Treating the Alcoholic: A Developmental Model of Recovery.* New York: Wiley.

Burkhalter, P. (1975). Alcoholism, drug abuse and drug addiction: A study of nursing education. *Journal of Nursing Education, 14*(2), 30–36.

Einstein, S., & Wolfson, E. (1970). Alcoholism curriculum: How professionals are trained. *International Journal of the Addictions, 5*(2), 295–312.

Ferneau, E., Jr., & Morton, E. (1968). Nursing personnel and alcoholism. *Nursing Research* (2), 174–177.

Kirkpatrick, J. (1986). *Turnabout: New help for the woman alcoholic.* Seattle: Madrona Publishers.

Mack, J. E. (1981). Alcoholism, A. A., and the governance of self. In M. Bean & N. Zinberg (Eds.), *Dynamic Approaches to the Understanding and Treatment of Alcoholism* (pp. 128–162). New York: The Free Press.

National Nurses Society on Addictions. (1987, March). *National survey of impaired nurse programs.* Evanston, IL: Author.

Vaillant, G. (1983). *Natural history of alcoholism.* Cambridge and London: Harvard University Press.

Zimberg, S., Wallace, J., & Blume, S. (Eds.). (1978). *Practical approaches to alcoholism psychotherapy.* New York: Plenum Press.

Appendix of Self-Help Groups

The following is a list of self-help groups that are especially relevant for impaired nurses. It is by no means exhaustive, but is included to aid readers in locating groups in their area.

Alcoholics Anonymous. Fellowship of men and women who share their experience, strength and hope with each other that they may solve their common problems and help each other recover from alcoholism. Started in 1935. 32,000 groups nationwide; 63,000 groups worldwide. Write: Box 459, Grand Central Station, New York, NY 10163. Call: (212) 686-1100. Local numbers listed in telephone directory.

Alanon Family Group. Designed to help family members and friends of problem drinkers by offering comfort, hope and friendship through sharing experience. Organized 1951. Over 22,000 groups worldwide. Write: PO Box 862, Midtown Station, New York, NY 10018-0862. Call: (212) 302-7240.

Alateen. Group for younger family members of alcoholics. Helps the young person learn to cope with the stress of living in an alcoholic family and to develop coping strategies. Organized in 1957. Over 3,000 chapters. Write: Alanon Family Group Headquarters listed above.

Calix Society. Association of Catholic Alcoholics maintaining sobriety through AA. Membership is not restricted to Catholics. Organized in 1947. About 58 chapters nationwide, 70+ chapters worldwide. Write: 7601 Wayzata Blvd., Minneapolis, MN 55426. Call: (612) 546-0544.

Cocaine Anonymous. Fellowship of men and women who share experience and strength to overcome addiction to cocaine. Organized 1982. Approximately 340 groups nationwide. Write: PO Box 1367, Culver City, CA 90232. Call: (213) 559-5833.

Emotions Anonymous. Fellowship of persons who share experience, strength and hope with each other so they may solve common problems of mental health. Organized 1968. 700 chapters nationwide, 1000 chapters worldwide. Write: PO Box 4245, St. Paul, MN 55104. Call: (612) 647-9712.

Impaired Nurse Network. The National Nurses Society on Addictions Impaired Nurse Committee maintains a network of contacts across the country that are available to assist nurses to contact resources. It helps nurses contact other nurses interested in the issue of nursing impairment as well as helping recovering nurses contact each other. Support groups for nurses are listed as well as individuals. The network may be utilized by contacting the Chairperson, Pat Green, at 1020 Sunset Drive, Lawrence, KS 66044. Telephone: (913) 842-3893.

J.A.C.S. (Jewish Alcoholics, Chemically Dependent Persons & Significant Others). For alcoholic and chemically dependent Jews, their families and their community. Organized 1980. 12 chapters. Write: 197 Broadway, Rm. M-7, New York, NY 10002. Call: (212) 473-4747.

Narcotics Anonymous. Fellowship of men and women who share their experience, strength and hope with each other that they may recover from drug addiction. Organized 1953. 5000 chapters worldwide. Write: PO Box 9999, Van Nuys, CA 92409. Call: (818) 780-3951.

Naranon Family Groups. Fellowship of family members and friends of persons dependent on drugs. Patterned after Alanon. Write: Naranon Family Group Headquarters, PO Box 2562, Palos Verdes, CA 92704. Call: (213) 547-5800.

National Association for Children of Alcoholics. Support and information for adult children of alcoholics. These groups recognize that growing up in an alcoholic home may leave emotional scars that will affect the person's life adversely unless recognized and addressed. Organized 1983. Write: NACOA, PO Box 421691, San Francisco, CA 94142.

Overeaters Anonymous. Fellowship of men and women who meet to help each other solve their common problems of compulsive overeating. Organized 1960. 7000 chapters nationwide. Write: 2190 W. 190th Street, Torrance, CA 90504.

Women for Sobriety. Program designed to meet the needs of female alcoholics. Emphasis placed on building self-esteem and assertiveness skills. Organized 1975. 350 chapters nationwide. Write: Box 618, Quakertown, PA 18951. Call: (215) 536-8026.

10

Reentering the Professional Practice Environment

Suzanne Durburg and June Werner

Probably the most common response to the nurse whose impairment can no longer be denied is dismissal. Because many chemically dependent nurses are outstanding caregivers, directors of nursing often have difficulty reporting them to the state board of nursing. It is easier to dismiss the nurse for failure to perform effectively. Such action sets a dangerous precedent, one that is difficult to correct. Most nurse executives have had experiences with addicted professionals who move from job to job because their nurse colleagues have not reported them to the state board. These chemically dependent nurses are often viewed as unfortunate persons burdened with an incurable moral malady.

Recent Views of Impairment

Only recently has the profession recognized that addiction and substance abuse are occupational hazards for nurses. The more common experience has been one of a conspiracy of silence on the part of colleagues accompanied by failure to view the problem as a treatable illness. This response has occurred largely because of lack of understanding about the addictive process. There is also a prevailing notion that nursing, as an extremely stressful profession, takes its toll on the personal lives of nurses, often leading them to manage these stressors with chemicals. In other words, nursing has developed a philosophical tolerance to drug and alcohol addiction as the logical consequence for some nurses of being continually under stress.

This point of view, as described above, holds little hope for anyone to intervene and to treat chemical addictions successfully. Once the colleagues of the addicted nurse are introduced to methods of intervention and treatment, the educational process and a more hopeful attitude can begin.

Only within the last decade has come the recognition by the profession that chemical dependency is a treatable illness. The concept of chemical dependency as a disease is now widely accepted (Talbott, Douglas, & Cooney, 1982) and is ascribed to by the authors. In 1982 the American Nurses' Association adopted a resolution urging the states to develop guidelines for peer-assistance programs. Endorsement by this professional organization has provided motivation and support to nurse executives striving for a more enlightened view of this problem and its treatment (ANA, 1984).

As in the days of Florence Nightingale, alcoholic and chemically dependent nurses work among us. Throughout the history of the profession, responses to the problem have ranged from denial, to punishment, to diagnosis of psychiatric illness, and finally to the promulgation of the disease concept. Alcoholism and drug addiction are primary illnesses. This understanding has brought hope and successful recovery to hundreds of nurses who formerly would have been lost from the profession (ANA, 1984).

Patient Safety Issues

In this era of cost reduction, early discharge, and concern over patients' length of hospital stay, one of the major responsibilities of nurse executives is to guarantee safe care to patients. The hospital or health care agency has a basic responsibility to provide safe care to its patients or clients. This is part of a covenant with the public, a moral and ethical promise that the institution must honor. This charge leads nurse executives to examine the broad issue of risk management. It is a priority for institutions facing an increasing number of malpractice cases and higher costs for malpractice coverage. Increasingly, hospitals have stiffened the requirements for malpractice coverage of staff physicians. They are also increasingly concerned about their liability for and the risks involved in managing nurses whose professional functioning is impaired. One need only recall concerned community response to media coverage of nurses or physicians diverting drugs from patients to realize that consumers want to have confidence in the people from whom they receive care (Beck & Buckley, 1983). This confidence can be destroyed when patients suffer as a result of nurse impairment. For example, patients receiving narcotic medication for pain control are at risk for denial of their required drug if they are cared for by a drug-addicted nurse. This nurse most frequently finds the unit's narcotic box the most accessible source of the drug. The addicted nurse either uses any excess narcotic herself or denies the patient prescribed pain medication. In some instances, nurses have substituted normal saline or water in prepackaged dose syringes. Fortunately, evidence of tampering is easily detected so that these contaminated drugs will not be used. Nonetheless, it is the real or potential threat of denying required medication to patients that makes it most difficult for fellow professionals to be sympathetic toward the addicted nurse, even though in the authors' experience, most recovering nurses claim to have diverted drugs that would otherwise have been discarded. It is therefore important that nurses record the results of any intervention they make to control their patient's pain. After the administration of any narcotic or analgesic, patient response to the pain medication should be recorded in the medical record. If the institution formally adopts this practice, it then becomes easier to identify patient-response patterns that point to a nurse who may be diverting drugs.

Professional Standards Issues

One of the hallmarks of the profession is its ability to set its own standards and hold its members accountable to them. As the nursing profession has become more established, efforts in this regard have become more formal. The American Nurses' Association has set standards for nursing practice and developed a code for nurses (ANA, 1985). Individual institutions also set performance expectations through the development of job descriptions, policies and procedures, quality assurance activities, and performance evaluations. These are most useful when expectations of performance are stated in clear, objective behavioral terms. Examples of inadequate or inappropriate performance frequently provide nurse managers with early evidence of the existence of a problem. Documentation of such events is also an important step in identifying nurses with chemical addiction. Once the performance problem is documented, efforts can be directed toward identifying the underlying cause. When consistently applied, well-developed standards of performance can provide a useful tool to nurse managers in the timely identification of chemically dependent nurses (AHA, 1985).

Why lose these valued employees? The impaired nurse, successfully treated and committed to recovery, provides to colleagues and the institution an example of victory over disease. The nurse has taken the opportunity for treatment and has been successful in the recovery process. The nurse's colleagues have had an opportunity to witness a story of personal tragedy and triumph and to learn a valuable lesson they may later apply in other circumstances. The institution saves dollars by preventing the loss of an experienced professional and has also raised the morale of other staff who view with approval and great satisfaction the fact that their employer provides a supportive environment for employees. This chapter presents issues of importance to the impaired nurse's reentry to practice.

Implementing Reentry

Once the addicted nurse has completed an initial treatment program, a careful assessment should be made prior to allowing the nurse to return to the work setting. Nurses should be assessed individually, but the nurse should certainly be protected from any exposure to controlled substances as opportunities for employment are evaluated. In some instances, nurses require a prolonged absence from the hospital setting in order to strengthen their position of recovery. Indeed for some nurses, return to nursing may not be recommended. Whatever the case, careful, individualized assessment should be made before the nurse returns to work.

The nurse who returns to her place of employment following rehabilitation faces many reentry challenges. While it is essential that confidentiality be maintained, safe effective reentry programs require that those supervising the recovering nurse be fully informed. Conditions of return to employment should be presented clearly to the nurse. They should include periodic, random drug screening tests, regular attendance at AA, NA, and other support groups, and regular, frequent performance appraisals. At times, nurses have found it supportive to their recovery to inform the staff on the unit where they resume employment of the nature of their impairment. Rather than promote or increase feelings of shame, recovering nurses report that sharing their situation with their colleagues can be a liberating experience. Other nurses seem to identify with their recovering peer and are anxious to provide support and encouragement for them. This attitude may explain why there has been minimal objection by staff to what may seem to be preferential treatment regarding scheduled day hours, with no shift rotation for the returning nurse. In any case, the environment to which the recovering nurse returns must be modified. Exposure to narcotics should be eliminated if possible. Whatever the role chosen for the returning nurse, the employer has the responsibility to screen carefully for the appropriateness of the role and its potential for adding or lessening stress on the job (Veatch, 1987).

Nurse managers should thoughtfully select an appropriate position to offer the returning nurse. Issues for consideration include the supportiveness of other staff on the unit, as well as the level of stress inherent in the position selected. Returning nurses should, if at all possible, not rotate shifts and should work day shift if possible. Protection of the public is paramount, even as the institution seeks to facilitate the recovery of the nurse. Performance expectations should be formulated into a contract (see Appendix A), which the nurse agrees to as a condition of reentry. A program for recovery is a lifelong commitment for the nurse. It is crucial it be expected as part of any reentry agreement. Some institutions have programs in place for recovering nurses that deal specifically with long-term professional recovery issues. If the institution has an effective Employee Assistance Counselor, that person may coordinate reentry expectations and monitor the nurse's progress. Under well-defined conditions such as these, the risk to an institution in rehiring a recovering nurse is minimal. Indeed some would agree that such a person is less of a risk than hiring a nurse who is unknown to the employer.

Case Histories

The authors have persuaded two recovering nurses to share their personal stories of addiction and recovery. Both nurses have continued their employment and contribute to patient care and outreach to other impaired colleagues. They are generous to tell their stories in an effort to educate and inform, and the authors are grateful for their participation.

Story A

I entered treatment after years of alcohol and drug abuse, culminating in severe addiction to intravenous narcotics, which I obtained illegally from work. I had managed to destroy my personal relationships and had nearly gotten myself fired (behavioral changes, tardiness, etc.). When I was confronted by supervisors, I was given a choice: terminate and be reported to the state licensing board or enter treatment. At this point, all I had left was my job and my license—what little self-esteem I had remaining was as a nurse. To lose my license meant to lose what was left of me. To me, there was no choice. It was over. So with shame and guilt engulfing me, I made the decision that changed my life. That same day I entered the hospital.

Because of insurance coverage restrictions, I could only be hospitalized at the institution that employed me for the past eight years. Initially I fought it, but ultimately I was too sick to put up too much of an argument. And, in true alcoholic fashion, I knew this was one way I could still maintain control. I knew the system, and I knew my way around. I was given a pseudonym to protect my anonymity, my name was different, but my face was the same. When doctors and other ancillary personnel came on the unit, I would make myself scarce. I expended an inordinate amount of energy hiding from people I knew. As I progressed in treatment, the shame abated ever so slightly, and I was able to face a few people I thought would not betray my confidence. When I was allowed "campus privileges," I would frequently run into some of my fellow staff nurses, often when I least expected it. Although difficult for me (and probably for them, also), these meetings spared me the fantasies of what I would say to these people and of the fear of rejection. Perhaps, though, the most advantageous part of hospitalization where I worked was the feeling of support from the staff, which continues to this day. Had I been hospitalized elsewhere, I wouldn't have the sense of rapport I have with these people. They know me, and I trust them, which is no small matter.

While still in treatment, I was guaranteed a job somewhere in the institution, although I remember being somewhat dubious about this promise. But they were true to their word and even respected my hesitancy toward working in the newborn or infant special care nursery. It was obvious, even to me, that I couldn't be allowed access to any drugs. A position opened in IV Therapy, and I was given the job. The irony did not escape me. When they told me I couldn't return to work for a month, I was furious. I felt I was being punished. As my recovery progressed, I was able to see that the people who were trying to help me knew what they were doing. If I'd gone back to work immediately, I would have done exactly what they were trying to prevent—using work as a means to avoid looking at myself.

Returning to the work force scared me to death—who knew about me? How would they react? Joining IV Therapy meant high visibility; I couldn't hide on one floor. The EAP Counselor advised me to be honest with the others in my new department as there was some speculation about my arrival. So I faced ten people I barely knew and gave them a brief rundown of what had happened. Expecting the worse (would they refuse to speak to me?), the reaction was one of respect. I was still paranoid about who in the institution knew, and I often read more into comments than was actually there. It took me a while to learn I was not the center of attention, that people had their own problems. So my fears decreased over time. I'm still working in this job, and this paranoia is nonexistent today.

The shame of addiction, especially for a nurse, is devastating. This is why I was so paranoid. I was lucky to have linked up with a very structured support group for recovering nurses as part of aftercare: This group dealt specifically with issues such as shame, guilt, the disease process—all problems addicts face. But for nurses, some of these feelings can be overwhelming. It was in this group I began to put to rest my shame and guilt. These feelings still surface occasionally, but I've learned to cope with them, and not let them get the better of me. I'm responsible for my recovery, not my disease.

This group did urine testing, on a random basis, in addition to reporting my progress in the group to the EAP Counselor. I was required to meet regularly with the counselor, and to continue seeing a therapist. I did as I was told, but felt as though big brother was watching. I understood the hospital must protect itself, and I knew I was very lucky they didn't toss me out on my ear, but the constant scrutiny was maddening. I may have been sick, but I was no fool—I went along with it.

The urine screens were the single, most motivating factor in keeping me sober. I must stress that, in my case, I did not get clean for myself. Although I felt guilty that I did it mainly to keep my license, I was also terrified as I knew that wasn't enough to keep me sober. I needed those urine screens. Any time I had the desire or opportunity to use, all I had to do was think of the monitoring. The fear of retribution kept me honest. I laugh now, at the story I can tell, without fear, of how I told myself I'd stay clean for a year, keep "them" happy, but when that year was up. . . . But when that year was up, I was finally clean and sober for myself, and I no longer needed those threats of urine testing. Today I don't use because of choice, not fear. This is not to say I don't think about it anymore—I do. But I remember well what the disease, in its active state, did to me. I don't want to live that life anymore.

I have many reasons to stay clean now, not the least of which is the trust my colleagues and supervisors have in me. I am keenly aware of being projected as a role model of a recovering nurse. I know that should I relapse, I would not only gravely disappoint myself but those who bent over backwards for me. In my support group, I was the only RN who was not fired for diverting. I know they went out on a limb for me. I'm proud of myself, and I'm proud of the nursing administrators for their progressive and non-judgmental attitude.

I am no longer monitored, and I don't have "big brother" hovering over me anymore. This is as it should be. I've come a long way from being a sick, addicted nurse, close to death, to one who is now able to help others who are ill. Much of the credit for this must go to those who understand that addiction to alcohol and drugs is a disease and to the people who saw in me a life worth saving, and, when I least expected it, offered compassion, respect, and hope. They have my everlasting gratitude.

Story B

Completion of an inpatient treatment program for chemical dependency provided me with the foundation upon which my recovery is based. In treatment, I learned that I could choose whether or not to use drugs and alcohol. I had lost my freedom of choice in the active stage of my addiction. I did not want to use, but was terrified that I could not survive and be at peace with myself without drugs. Drugs helped me to like me. Treatment taught me that I could live without drugs. I was able to tolerate living and reality without resorting to a chemical, and I was beginning to feel better about me.

I honestly was not ceratin that I would ever practice nursing again. There was a good deal of uncertainty at the hospital where I was employed as to what to do with me. At times I felt as if they would be happier if I quit. I was ambivalent about returning. A part of me wanted to avoid the people with whom I had worked. Another part of me knew I had to face them, as I had been hiding in my addiction for too long. I was experiencing so much shame.

While on an intellectual level, I believed that chemical dependency was a disease, I felt that I was the only nurse to whom this had ever happened and believed myself to be morally weak. I felt that as a nurse I should have known better.

I was very much alone in the early days of my recovery. After completing treatment, I was off work an additional month. This was done to provide me with some time to take care of me and get my recovery program into place. We nurses are very good at taking care of everyone else at the expense of ourselves. It was much easier for me to look at others' problems versus looking at mine. The hospital where I work felt that this time was important to my recovery. At the time I felt that it was punitive. In retrospect, I am grateful that they cared enough about me to give me the time.

During this time off work, I was attending daily self-help group meetings, attending an aftercare support group weekly at the treatment center, seeing my therapist twice a week, and in contact with the Employee Assistance Program director. My motivation at this time was purely to retain my nursing license (I had been reported to the Department of Registration and Education while in treatment). I had not yet begun to reap the benefits of living a chemically free life. I did, however, know and accept that drugs and nursing did not mix.

It was decided that I could return to work, but it had to be in an area with little or no narcotic use. My love was orthopedics. I could understand not returning there immediately because so many narcotics were dispensed. I could understand, but I didn't have to like it. I was convinced that I would be working in the nursery or housekeeping—neither of which was particularly appealing. However, I was determined to accept where I was placed and attempt to make it work. I had made a decision to try it their (the hospital's) way because my way hadn't worked. I would have done anything asked of me.

I met with Nurse Recruitment and was shocked at how kind they were to me. They did not treat me like a moral degenerate and worked at finding a place for me. At some point during this time, I began to believe that the disease concept of chemical dependency applied to me. I was not a bad nurse, but rather a sick nurse working on getting well.

I accepted a position on the Infant Special Care Unit. My confidentiality was respected, but I was told that it was important that certain people working on my unit needed to be told my history. This included the Clinical Director, Clinical Coordinator, and three nurses who oriented me. It was up to me if I chose to tell anyone else. At the time I returned to work, I agreed to have random urine samples taken for drug screening. I found this to be extremely supportive to my recovery.

I began a ten-week orientation. It was decided that I could not administer any mood-altering substance for a three-month period, and no controlled substance for a period of six months. The small amounts of phenobarbital and chloral hydrate that we gave the babies were administered by the nurses orienting me. I completed the ten-week orientation period in seven weeks. I continued with my recovery program, as outlined earlier, but cut back the self-help group meetings to three to four per week.

I was beginning to feel good about myself and my recovery. Those who knew of my history were very accepting and supportive of me. I also, during this time, began to receive phone calls from those I had worked with on orthopedics, expressing their support. This helped the healing process. Because others could accept me and my disease, I could accept me and my disease. I could begin to forgive myself and the shame began to lessen.

The random urine samples continued. The message I had received upon returning to work was that if a urine turned up positive for drugs, I would be terminated. This limit was necessary. Drug addicts and alcoholics need limits because we can always find the loophole. This limit eliminated any thoughts I may have had about using. Nursing was too important to me.

About two months after I returned to work, I received a phone call from the Employee Assistance Director, asking me to come into his office before going to work. I did not like the whole feel of this call. I was feeling extremely anxious and spent a good deal of time trying to determine what I had done, as this was not the time for my usual appointment. I had nothing to hide or be ashamed of, but I still had this uneasy feeling. I went to the hospital early. Sitting in the office were the Clinical Coordinator, the Clinical Director, and Associate Chairman of the Department of Nursing and the Director of EAP. The lab report of my drug screen was being handed out, and it had turned up positive for morphine! I was clean, but they had no reason in the world to believe me. I was terminated on the spot, and further treatment was offered.

I was furious. I was living a drug-free life, doing the right things, and feeling better about me, but they chose to believe the lab. I knew that it was a lab error and decided to pursue this and prove my innocence. My therapist was the only one who believed me, and supported my pursuing this.

I contacted the Director of the lab and asked that the drug screen be rerun. The specimen, which should have been kept for two weeks, had disappeared. I made some phone calls to attorneys and to the EAP. The EAP asked me not to do anything further until he got back to me, as they were looking into it at the hospital. My Clinical Director had apparently believed me and pursued this herself. She discovered that the validity of the drug screen was 50%. Meanwhile, it was discovered that my urine had been taken to a toxicology class and run on a new machine. The urine specimen was clean. I was reinstated and received an apology.

This was a difficult time for me. I look at this as a test of my recovery. Not one time during this period did I think of using drugs. I was finally feeling comfortable with me and my recovery. I had come to accept that drugs would only make a bad situation a million times worse. This was new thinking for me. I was, and still am, constantly amazed that I could get through difficult times without drugs. I was beginning to feel comfortable with me and liking it.

I continued to work on the Infant Special Care Unit. After three months, I was allowed to administer chloral hydrate and phenobarbital. I found, however, that as much as I wanted this job to work, I was not getting the same satisfaction that I did working with adults on orthopedics. The agreement had been that I could not administer or be anywhere near controlled substances for at least six months. As my six-month anniversary approached, I requested a transfer back to orthopedics. There were many meetings regarding this. The powers that be, I suspect, felt that it was too soon, and that I was setting myself up. However, they agreed to the transfer and set up guidelines for my administering narcotics.

I returned to orthopedics with the following guidelines in place: (1) for the first two weeks a designated nurse co-signed narcotics with me and accompanied me to the bedside to administer them; (2) all wastes had to adhere to hospital policy, i.e., be witnessed and co-signed appropriately; and (3) the frequency of random urine samples increased. These stipulations were agreeable to me as they provided me with additional support and limits. I was also returning to a work setting where my colleagues knew me when I was sickest, but at the same time had been there for me as I struggled through my early days of recovery. I wanted recovery at this point, but I also did not want to let them down. I wanted to earn back their trust and respect. I felt safe in this environment. This is not to say that I was not fearful. The question foremost in my mind was will the obsession and compulsion that I had lived with every time I opened the narcotic box be gone? When I opened that box for the first time, my hands shook, but the obsession and compulsion were gone. I was able to function as a more effective and respected professional. This is not to say that I had no thoughts of using—I did, and occasionally still do. However, I have learned more effective means of dealing with the problems of living and the daily stresses of our profession. Thinking about drugs and acting on those thoughts are two different things.

At approximately the same time that I was returning to orthopedics, the Department of Registration and Education of the State of Illinois contacted me regarding a report they had received concerning me and the diversion of narcotics from the hospital where I was, and continue to be, employed. I was given the option of appearing before the Board of Nurse Examiners or accepting the chief prosecutor's recommendation. I opted for the latter. A meeting was set up with the investigator and those at the hospital who had made the complaint, but at the same time, were supportive of my recovery. Approximately one month later, I received the outcome and recommendations. I was placed on probation for a period of five years. If during this five-year period I returned to drug use, my license would be suspended for one year. I was required to provide the Department of Registration and Education with documentation, as they requested it, of my continued efforts at sobriety (including drug screens, if requested). If I changed my place of employment, I was required to notify the department of the change and the reason for leaving my job. I viewed this as supportive and was grateful to have my nursing license intact.

I continued to work on orthopedics until I was chemically free for two years. During this time, I made myself available to the Employee Assistance Program should another nurse dependent on alcohol or drugs want to talk with me. I did not want anyone else to feel as alone as I did in the early days of my recovery. I had so much gratitude to those in my profession who cared about me when I was so sick. My recovery teaches me that I have to give to someone else that which I have received. In doing this, I feel that it has helped me deal with the shame I experienced in the early days and to some extent into the present.

As a result of my work with other chemically dependent nurses, I became interested in working on the chemical-dependency unit at my hospital. I was offered a job there two years into my recovery and continue to work there. This job has given me many opportunities to grow. It also gives me a daily reminder of where I will be if I become complacent in my recovery program. I have had the opportunity to work with many other chemically dependent nurses. I have been involved in educating our profession about the impaired nurse. Recently, a few other nurses and I began a support group for the impaired nurse.

If I had not recovered from the disease of chemical dependency, I would not be writing this today. I was slowly dying. I did not have a choice of using drugs or not using drugs—I had to use. I was a prisoner of my disease. Today I have the freedom of choice. I am not imprisoned by my disease. I have to remember on a daily basis that I am a drug addict and an alcoholic before I am anything else. I have to work on me to keep my disease in remission. There is no cure for addiction. I was sick for a very long time on physical, emotional, and spiritual levels, and it takes time to heal. I have to work on patience. I have to work on perfectionism, and acceptance that I'm human and by definition imperfect. I have to work on being comfortable with this. I have slowly come to be at peace with myself. I looked to drugs for peace in the past. Today I look to other people and my recovery program for peace. In the past, I attempted to control reality and my feelings with chemicals. Today I can accept that it is all right to feel. I didn't always believe this. I am grateful to my friends, my family, and my profession for caring about me when I didn't care about me. I am grateful to be living the life I am today.

The Role of the Nurse Executive

Chemical dependency among nurses will not disappear. Drug and alcohol abuse and addiction has become recognized as a significant problem in the United States, and its existence in the nursing profession must be acknowledged. The nursing profession is under great pressure to control, if not eliminate, drug use among nurses. However, we will fail if we take a punitive and dogmatic approach to the problem.

The nurse executive plays a pivotal role in any institution's seeking to develop an enlightened and effective approach to nurse impairment. It is imperative that nurse executives understand the addictive process and the successful outcomes of a rehabilitative approach based on this view.

Educating Hospital Leadership

The governing board of a health care institution expects the nurse executive to be accountable for delivery of safe, competent, high quality nursing care to its patients. The well-informed nurse executive should, therefore, apprise the hospital administrator and human resources department of the potential existence of impairment among the nursing staff. The nurse executive may be reluctant to acknowledge that impairment exists. Such denial is not easily sustained, however, for the nurse executive will inevitably be confronted with the problem (O'Connor & Robinson, 1985). In the role of nursing staff advocate, the nurse executive has a major responsibility to educate other administrators and executives at the institution about the problem of impairment among nurses. It is also useful to present a clinical perspective on the disease of chemical dependency and the successful treatment outcomes of those who sought treatment. It is of the utmost importance that nonclinical hospital executives accept the disease concept, so that they will support and approve this approach to the management of impaired employees. The nurse executive may find it advantageous to present the problem as one shared by the physicians as well. Nurses and physicians working together with hospital administration may prove more effective in receiving support for the rehabilitative approach to the problem of professional impairment. Jointly sponsored educational programs can be useful in educating the hospital's professional community about the problem.

Developing Procedures to Deal With Impairment

Once the nurse executive has succeeded in educating the leadership of the institution about the problem of nurse impairment, the development of policies and procedures for managing such a problem must occur. A well articulated, philosophical position should frame the policies and procedures that follow it. Acknowledgment that chemical dependency is a treatable disease should be central to any philosophical statement. Each institution can then individualize its approach based on its own value system at it applies to employee relations (see Appendix B).

The development of specific policies and procedures can be an arduous task. There are many concerns to be addressed at this point, including state regulations and reporting requirements, legal liability, hospital policies related to theft, the ever-present concern for patient safety, and community relations. If the institution has an Employee Assistance Counselor, the role of that professional should also be stated. Consequences of return to drug or alcohol use should be delineated, including reporting such an occurrence to the State Board of Nursing. A policy based on a model of rehabilitation should not be viewed as "lenient." Firm and unequivocal requirements that addicted nurses participate in specified treatment and recovery programs should be clearly stated and enforced.

An Employee Assistance Program can be a source of great support and assistance to nursing managers faced with the complex problem of impairment. A well informed and experienced Employee

Assistance Counselor can help direct activities of confrontation, intervention, and the selection of an appropriate treatment facility for the affected nurse. If one's own institution does not employ such a person, assistance can be gained from an outside consultant who can provide similar support. The Employee Assistance Counselor should provide continuity of care and support for the recovering nurse from the moment of identification through treatment and reentry and can assist in sustaining recovery.

Educating Hospital Staff

Once an institution has developed policies and procedures to respond to the issue of impaired professional functioning, it is important to take this information to the managers of the institution and to the staff nurses themselves. Educational programs by the Employee Assistance Counselor on the existence and treatment of chemical dependency should be presented to all nurse managers and staff nurses. This program should include information on the existence and scope of the problem and approaches to identification and performance evaluation, intervention, treatment, and reentry. This educational process can be reinforced by offering periodic programs with speakers on the issue of impairment among nurses. A most compelling and effective approach involves enlisting the help of recovering nurses to tell their own stories of addiction and recovery.

Peer Review

The implementation of an effective peer review program as part of an evaluation process for staff nurses as well as nurses in administrative and other leadership positions is necessary to meet the professional responsibility we have to each other and to consumers. An effective peer-review program creates an atmosphere in which nurses provide regular, honest responses to each other's performance in a helpful, structured and clearly documented fashion. A professional practice climate that includes peer review legitimizes the professional responsibilities nurses have but may be reluctant to implement. It can be threatening to confront dysfunctional behavior in one's colleagues unless the system in which one works provides a framework for airing and acting on such information. Peer review is not a panacea, but assisting nurses to develop effective skills in evaluating each other's performance may create an environment less conducive to enabling behaviors.

The need for competent nurses has increased. The present nursing shortage is projected to intensify (AONE, 1986). The nursing profession would be wise to identify more vigorously those among us who are impaired and to facilitate the recovery process so that they may continue to provide patient care. The present estimates of the incidence of impairment among nurses point to our pressing obligation as professionals to identify and assure our colleagues access to treatment.

References

American Hospital Association. (1985). *American hospital association hospital employee assistance programs.* Chicago: Author.

American Hospital Association. (December, 1986). American Organization of Nurse Executives, Report of the 1986 Hospital Nursing Supply, Unpublished Survey.

American Nurses' Association. (1984). *Addictions and psychological dysfunctions in nursing: The profession's response to the problem.* Kansas City, MO: Author.

American Nurses' Association, (1985). *Code for nurses.* Kansas City, MO: Author.

Beck, M., & Buckley, J. (1983). "Nurses With Bad Habits." *Newsweek,* August 22, p. 54.

O'Connor, P., & Robinson, R. S. (1985). Managing impaired nurses." *Nursing Administration Quarterly, 9(2), 1–9.*

Talbott, G. D., & Cooney, M. (1982). Today's disease alcohol drug dependence, Springfield, IL: Charles C. Thomas.

Veatch, D. (1987). "When is the recovering impaired nurse ready to work. A job interview guide." *Journal of Nursing Administration,* 17(2), 14–16.

Appendix A

Reentry Contract for the Recovering Nurse

I __________ acknowledge that I suffer from the disease of alcoholism and/or chemical dependency, and agree to the following as conditions of my continued employment for a period of ______;

1. To abstain completely from alcohol and any mood-altering drugs or chemicals;
2. To actively and consistently participate in a program of recovery which includes attendance at Alcoholics Anonymous and/or Narcotics Anonymous, the Recovering Nurses' Group, and any other activities as directed by the Employee Assistance Counselor;
3. To voluntarily submit to random urine testing, with the understanding that if a result is positive, I may be terminated and reported to the State Board of Nursing;

4. To maintain my job performance at satisfactory levels, and to participate in regular performance evaluations as required.

Recovering Nurse Employee Assistance Counselor

Vice President, Nursing

Appendix B*

Subject: Fitness for Duty

1. POLICY
   Our policies and guidelines for appropriate employee behavior are predicated on patient care needs and quality of care standards. Accordingly, along with this management philosophy is our responsibility to fulfill our fiduciary responsibility with regard to the safe and efficient operation of the Hospitals for all persons. For these reasons, and out of concern for the well being of our employees, Evanston Hospital Corporation has developed this policy regarding employee fitness for duty.

   The Evanston Hospital Corporation is strongly committed to promoting employee health and maintaining a safe environment for patients, visitors, and employees that is free of the effects of alcohol and drug use and abuse and inappropriate employee behavior. Consistent with this commitment, employees are required to report for work and perform their jobs appropriately and without any adverse effects due to the use or abuse of any drug, medication, or alcohol, as defined below.

**Source:* Evanston Hospital, 2650 Ridge Avenue, Evanston, IL 60201.

While the Hospital has no intention of unnecessarily intruding into the private lives of its employees, the Hospital does expect employees to report for work in a mental and physical condition to be able to perform their duties safely and efficiently. It must be recognized that off the job as well as on the job use of legal and illegal drugs and alcohol by employees can have an unacceptable impact on workplace safety and productivity and interfere with the Hospital's goal of maintaining a safe environment that is free of the adverse effects of alcohol and drug use and abuse. This, in turn, would affect the Hospitals's ability to provide safe health care services to its patients.

2. PURPOSE

The purpose of this policy is to assist employees who display inappropriate behavior, are mentally and physically unable to perform their job, or who may be chemically dependent. The Hospital's goal is to maintain a work environment free of the adverse effects of these problems.

Employees who violate this policy are subject to the employee conduct and termination policies. The Hospital shall provide a training program to educate managers and supervisors in recognizing inappropriate behavior and substance use or abuse situations as manifested in the workplace to encourage treatment before violations of Hospital policies might occur.

3. DEFINITION

For the purpose of this policy the terms listed below are defined as follows:

A. *Drug*—any over-the-counter medication; prescribed medication; illegal or unprescribed controlled chemical substance; or alcoholic beverage.

B. *Inappropriate Behavior/Under the Influence*—occurs whenever an employee is acting or behaving in a manner not suitable for the workplace or affected by drugs in any detectable manner, including, but not limited to, misconduct or obvious impairment of physical or mental ability. This can be established by a layperson's opinion as well as by a professional opinion or a scientifically valid test that the employee's blood alcohol concentration is .05 or greater, or in the case of illegal drugs, that there is any detectable presence of drug metabolites in an employee. (Illegal drug means any drug which is not legally obtainable and includes marijuana).

4. PROHIBITED CONDUCT

   The use, possession, sale, transfer, or exchange of drugs or reporting to work or being under the influence of drugs during working hours or while on the Hospital premises or while in a Hospital vehicle is prohibited, except as provided by paragraph five below, and employees are subject to Hospital Policy 3.06, "Guidelines for Employee Conduct" and Hospital Policy 3.11, "Involuntary Termination."

5. PROTOCOL

   A. All employees must notify the Employee Health Service when they are using over-the-counter or prescribed medication that they have been told or have reason to believe may affect their ability to perform their job. Employees may continue to work if the Employee Health Service has determined that the employee's drug use does not pose a safety threat and that the employee's job performance is not significantly affected. If use of the medication would affect the employee's job performance, the employee may be transferred, assigned different duties, or in some cases required to take sick time, if available, or a leave of absence for the duration of the use of the drug.

   B. The Hospital maintains an Employee Assistance Program (EAP) which provides confidential assistance to employees who suffer from alcohol or drug abuse and other personal/emotional problems. An integral and essential part of the Fitness for Duty policy is the EAP which is intended to help employees identify alcohol or drug problems and enter appropriate rehabilitation and counseling programs. The EAP also provides appropriate follow-up support. It is the responsibility of each employee to voluntarily seek assistance from the Employee Assistance Program before alcohol and drug problems lead to disciplinary action which may include termination for a first offense. In situations where violations of Hospital policy have not occurred, but where there is suspicion of drug or alcohol use, employees will be referred to the EAP for evaluation in an effort to avoid disciplinary action, if possible under the circumstances.

6. DRUG AND ALCOHOL TESTING
   The Hospital may require at any time a blood test, urinalysis, or other drug/alcohol test of any employee suspected of using or being under the influence of any drug or alcohol or whenever circumstances or workplace conditions may otherwise justify such a test. An employee's consent to submit to such a test is required as a condition of employment. A refusal to consent to such a test will result in termination of the employee.
7. SEARCHES
   Searches of employees' personal property may be conducted according to Hospital Policy 3.06, "Guidelines for Employee Conduct."

11

Evaluation of Treatment Outcome

Janet Gaskin

Purpose of Evaluation

The purpose of evaluation is to measure the effects of a program against the goals it set out to accomplish, in order to make decisions about future programming. The type and extent of the evaluation will be influenced by these goals or expectations. There are many reasons for deciding to evaluate a program, and these must be clearly identified at the outset and may include the need to decide whether or not to continue a program, to determine whether or not improvements are called for, and to determine whether or not to institute the same program elsewhere or to increase financial support for an existing program.

The two main types of evaluation are formative evaluation, which means that the criteria for evaluating a program guide or dictate the way in which the program is developed, and summation evaluation, wherein the evaluation is planned and designed once the program is finished. This distinction may not be useful, however, as some programs are ongoing.

Project Turnabout was a pilot project established in 1983 to determine whether or not there was a need for a specialized treatment program for nurses who had problems with drug and alcohol abuse in Ontario. It was essentially a needs-assessment pilot project.

A treatment system was set up by this author utilizing existing resources and facilities of the Clinical Institute, Addiction Research Foundation. In addition to proposing and initiating the project, the writer functioned as one of three primary care nurses.

Nurses wishing assistance contacted Project Turnabout by calling a 24-hr hotline, or they were referred by other sources in the community, including family, physician, or employer. The treatment process was explained to the nurse on the telephone and an intake appointment was made if appropriate.

The initial contact was with a nurse primary-care worker who assessed the client. After establishing a beginning relationship, the primary-care worker collected necessary demographic information. This information concerned employment status, legal problems, current and past drug use, past treatment experience, financial problems, extent of family and other social support, source of referral, health status, and the client's perception of the problem (see Appendices A, B, C, D). Treatment options were discussed with the client and an appropriate choice made. Treatment options included individual therapy for three to four months; group therapy on a weekly basis for six months; or intensive three-week-long day or residential programs. These options were used alone or in combination. The primary-care worker remained the case coordinator, or contact person, throughout that client's treatment. The client was contacted by the primary-care worker at least every three months for a period of 18 months. Initially, and at each contact, follow-up information was collected and progress documented.

Two research tools were used in an attempt to gather objective data. Both were administered at intake. The Inventory of Drinking/Drug Use Situations (IDS; Annis 1984; Annis, Graham, & Davis, 1987) is a 42-item questionnaire designed to identify situations in which an individual drank heavily or abused drugs in the past year. The items of the questionnaire are designed to assess eight situational categories of potential relapse divided into two major classes: (1) personal states, in which drinking or drug abuse involves a response to an event that is primarily psychological or physical in nature; and (2) situations involving other people, in which the influence of another person is significant. Personal states are further subdivided into five categories: negative emotional states (4 items); negative physical states (4 items); positive emotional states (4 items); testing personal control (4 items), and urges and temptations (4 items). Situations involving other people are subdivided into three categories: interpersonal conflict (12 items), social pressure to drink (4 items) and positive emotional states (6 items) (see Appendix E).

The second tool used is called the Situational Confidence Questionnaire (SCQ; Annis & Graham, 1987), a 42-item questionnaire designed to assess Bandura's concept of self-efficacy (Bandura, 1978) in relation to a client's perceived ability to cope effectively with alcohol and other drugs. The 42 items parallel the 42 situations employed in the Inventory of Drinking or Drug Use Situations (IDS). As with the IDS, the eight-category classification system derived from the work of Marlatt and his associates is employed to categorize high-risk drinking areas. (Marlatt, 1985a, b, c) (See Appendix F).

The SCQ was administered to all clients at intake and again after 6 months of treatment with the aim of identifying high-risk situations that may prompt a major relapse. However, no significant differences were found between scores at intake, and at six months. In addition, the majority of test scores indicate that these nurses are very confident at intake they will not abuse drugs or alcohol in any situation. However, considering the nurses are in a treatment program for substance abuse when this questionnaire is completed, this result may more likely reflect their need to believe treatment will be successful. Thus, for the purposes of evaluation the SCQ no longer had an apparent viable application.

The Evaluation Process

Essentially, the task of evaluators is to identify program goals, translate them into measurable parameters, collect data, and then compare the program's achievements with these goals. This seemingly straight-forward task is usually complicated by numerous factors, some of which are discussed below.

Program goals must be clearly stated in order to facilitate subsequent evaluation. Goals may be covert as well as overt, and short-as well as long-term. It is important to set measurable program goals. For example, one goal might be that clients will be able to return to work and perform satisfactorily. Choosing a goal of abstinence from drug use is less useful as it cannot be too reliably measured on a daily basis over time.

It is also important that the tools for measuring the extent to which program goals have been met must be carefully chosen in order to yield meaningful data. Usually, multiple measures are required for successful evaluation. These may include measures of knowledge, attitudes, behavior, and work performance, as well as financial costs. Data measuring knowledge and attitudes are less valuable in the evaluation of treatment programs than those measuring behavior changes, since most treatment programs endeavor to change behavior.

It is also important to consider variations within a given program; not every client in a program has the same treatment experience. For example, there are experienced and inexperienced therapists, same and both sex groups, individual and group therapy.

There are, then, two sets of variables at the outset; one set has to do with the program and the other includes client characteristics. There are also intervening variables that influence outcome, such as those which relate to program operation, e.g., staff turnover.

In order to demonstrate the effectiveness of Project Turnabout in reaching its goals, data were collected before treatment began, and at three-month intervals following treatment, for a period of eighteen months. The data included employment status, drug use, and the extent of involvement in the treatment process. A questionnaire addressing these issues was completed at each interval by the nurse primary-care worker. These outcomes were summarized and mean scores obtained for each item, thus enabling us to know, for example, what percentage of our clients were employed by the same employer 18 months after initiation of treatment.

Evaluation Designs

One of the most common evaluation designs can be diagrammed as follows: premeasure, treatment, postmeasure.

This is a descriptive, nonexperimental design. The decision regarding which data to collect at the premeasure stage must be made carefully. Sources for such data must include the client, family members, employers, or carefully chosen data collection instruments. Postmeasure data may also include observations or program records. Information obtained from this type of data, however, cannot be generalized, as the outcomes cannot be attributed to the program alone. The Project Turnabout evaluation design was of this type.

Quasi-experimental designs involve multiple groups. These may be groups of different types of clients or groups who receive different treatment. Examples of these types include time series, multiple time series, and nonequivalent control group designs. The major task is to control relevant outside effects.

True experimental design involves the use of experimental and control groups, as well as random assignment to these groups. The control group may receive no treatment, which can pose ethical problems, or they may receive the standard treatment, while the experimental group receives the experimental treatment. Obviously, the experimental treatment, from an ethical standpoint, must have some likelihood of doing good. Randomization effectively rules out the possibility that some factor other than the treatment has produced the desired outcome, e.g.,maturation or changes in the cultural environment. Randomization, then, is the essential requirement of a true experiment.

The true controlled experiment is often not possible in program evaluation, however. Many problems may arise, such as lack of sufficient subjects, wide geographic distribution of clients, resistance to random assignment by referral agents, contamination of the control group, the Hawthorne effect, and emotional reactions of clients who are accepted into the program. Nonetheless, where decisions about a program's continuation are to be made and a high level of confidence in results is essential, experimental design should be used.

Regardless of the design used for evaluation, the rights of the clients must be protected. Informed consent is necessary and must include detailed explanation and assurance of confidentiality to the client. In programs that deal with highly stigmatized behaviors such as drug abuse, these assurances may well determine whether or not a program is fully subscribed.

Evaluation of Project Turnabout

During the period from November 1983 to November 1986, 150 nurses were seen in Project Turnabout. At the end of this period, it was concluded that a separate treatment capability for nurses was indeed necessary and the "Project" was reestablished and funded as an incorporated entity, separate and apart from the Addiction Research Foundation.

The evaluation design was descriptive, nonexperimental, consisting of a premeasure and a postmeasure. Such studies can be useful in providing insights that will improve the operations of a program. Clearly, however, they fail to control for alternative explanations of behavioral changes, e.g., maturation, external events, etc. Therefore, these results must be viewed with caution and it must be recognized that these findings cannot be generalized to other programs.

Some exploratory research was begun during the pilot phase of the project. This included a comparison between demographic variables from a sample of nurses in Project Turnabout and a sample of female clients from similar occupational groups who presented for treatment of drug and alcohol abuse at the Addiction Research Foundation, during the same period (see Table 11.1).

Several questions have emerged for us from the data presented. They will be presented separately as follows.

Are nurses different from other female clients in comparable occupations with regard to reported substance of abuse? In order to explore this question further we obtained similar data for all female clients classified as having high status occupations who presented for treatment at Addiction Research Foundation in 1985 (see Table 11.2).

The most apparent difference between the nurse-sample and the nonnurse sample is the type of drug abused. The nurses have reported a much higher incidence of narcotic use (23%) than did the other group (10.7%). The nonnurse group revealed a greater reported abuse of alcohol in combination with other drugs (14.1% of sample) compared with the nurses in Project Turnabout (6%). The second

TABLE 11.1 Project Turnabout: Summary of Data on All Clients Who Entered the Program Between November '83–March '86. Description of the Sample at Intake ($N=100$)

Category	Percentage
Professional status	
RN's	82
RNA's	18
Source of referral	
Self-referrals	62
Employer referrals	26
Other	12
Employment status	
Employed	72
College of nurses involvement	18
Substance of abuse:	
Alcohol only	59
Opiate narcotics only	23
Other drugs (including benzodiazapam)	12
Alcohol and drugs	6

question we asked was whether the nurses in our sample who abused alcohol were different from their colleagues who abused other drugs. The instrument we chose to use to examine this question was the Inventory of Drinking/Drug Using Situations.

Analysis of the data from this questionnaire showed two significant differences between these two subsets of our nurse sample. The nurses who abused drugs other than alcohol scored significantly higher ($p<0.01$) on the subscale "negative physical states" (e.g., pain) than did the nurses who abused alcohol. This means that the drug-abusing subset reported using drugs more frequently in response to unpleasant bodily sensations or discomforts. This of course is a socially acceptable reason for narcotic analgesic use.

The nurses who abused alcohol scored significantly higher ($p<0.003$) on the subscale "social pressure to drink" than did the comparison group of nurses who abused drugs other than alcohol. This is also not a surprising finding as it is more socially acceptable

TABLE 11.2 Females with High Status Ocupations (*N*=72)

Category	Percentage
Source of referral	
Self	62.2
Employer	5.2
Legal	3.5
Other (family, doctor, hospital)	29.1
Employment status	
Employed	61.6
Unemployed	38.3
Substance of abuse	
Alcohol only	65.1
Narcotics	10.7
Other drugs	10.1
Alcohol and drugs	14.1

to report heavy drinking in the context of a social situation where there is overt or implicit pressure to drink alcohol.

We then sought to discover whether our sample of nurses who abused alcohol scored differently on the Inventory of Drinking Situations than nonnurse females who abused alcohol. For the purpose of this comparison we used a subsample of all females presenting for treatment of alcohol abuse at the Addiction Research Foundation between 1982 and 1984. This group was comprised of females from many different occupations. Table 11.3 presents this comparison.

A high mean score is interpreted as greater frequency of heavy drinking associated with situations included in that category in the past year, according to the client. As can be seen from Table 11.3, the nurse sample scored significantly lower on all elements of the Inventory of Drinking Situations when compared with other female alcohol abusers seeking treatment. This means that the alcohol-abusing nonnurse females reported significantly more situations on all subscales in which they drank heavily over the past year.

Discussion

It would seem that the sample of nurses we have seen in this unique treatment program is different from the two comparison groups of female clients. One difference is that a higher percentage of the nurse

TABLE 11.3 Project Turnabout Alcohol Users vs. General Groups of Female Alcohol Users[a]

IDS Subscale	Project turnabout clients (mean) (*N*=24)	Other female clients (mean) (*N*=45)
Intrapersonal determinants		
1. Negative emotional states	51.48	71.87
2. Negative physical states	35.72	56.78
3. Positive emotional states	31.64	58.31
4. Testing personal control	40.88	59.83
5. Urges and temptations	33.51	58.21
Interpersonal determinants		
1. Interpersonal conflict	35.91	60.68
2. Social pressure to drink	33.35	61.77
3. Positive emotional states	33.33	62.70

[a]Significance level=0.001.

sample reported narcotic abuse. It is possible that access to narcotics is a major factor influencing this finding. As a preventive strategy, measures to control access to narcotics more effectively are advisable. Nurses may also select narcotics due to the greater degree of knowledge they may have about drug effects. We would recommend educational programs for nurses regarding the abuse potential of narcotics combined with training in alternative measures for managing stress or emotional problems. These initiatives may decrease narcotic abuse by nurses.

Another area of difference is in the Inventory of Drinking Situations data where we find that nurses who presented for treatment of alcohol abuse reported significantly fewer situations in which they drank heavily prior to entering treatment.

This could mean that nurses do indeed have fewer situations in which they drink heavily or it could mean that these nurses drink less in all situations than the comparison group of other females. It could also be evidence of nurses' unwillingness to present an accurate picture of their drinking due to the negative impact this might have on their professional self-image. It is considered less acceptable for any female in our culture to drink heavily than for males.

On a subjective level, nurses appear to be very ashamed of their alcohol and drug abuse because it conflicts with their image of the professional nurse. These clients identify strongly with this image and thus their drug abuse may produce serious intrapsychic conflict for them.

Recommendations for Future Evaluations

More formal attempts to evaluate this program could be instituted now that the needs-assessment work is completed. Future evaluation research might use a true experimental design with random assignment to different treatment models. This might include inpatient versus outpatient, group versus individual, same-sex therapist versus opposite-sex therapist, nurse therapist versus nonnurse therapist, and mandatory versus voluntary treatment. Little is known about these variables in relation to nurses and treatment for substance abuse.

Clearly, a formative evaluation approach is ideal, where the program is designed with the evaluation process built in from the outset. The motivation or reason for the evaluation will, to a significant extent, dictate its final scientific quality.

References

Annis, H.M. (1984). *Inventory of drinking situations.* Toronto: Addiction Research Foundation of Ontario.

Annis, H.M., Graham, J.M., & Davis, C.S. (1987). *Inventory of drinking situations user's guide.* Toronto: Addiction Research Foundation.

Annis, H.M., & Graham, J.M. (1988). *Situational confidence questionnaire user's guide.* Toronto: Addiction Research Foundation.

Bandura, A. (1977). Reflections on self-efficacy. *Advances in Behavioral Research and Therapy, 1,* 237–269.

Marlatt, G. A. (1985a). Situational determinants of relapse and skill-training interventions. In G. A. Marlatt & J. R. Gordon (Eds.), *Relapse prevention: Maintenance strategies in the treatment of addictive behaviors.* New York: Guilford.

Marlatt, G.A. (1985b). Cognitive factors in the relapse process. In G.A. Marlatt & J.R. Gordon (Eds.) *Relapse prevention: Maintenance strategies in the treatment of addictive behaviors.* New York: Guilford.

Marlatt, G.A. (1985c). Cognitive assessment and intervention procedures for relapse prevention. In G.A. Marlatt & J.R. Gordon (Eds.), *Relapse prevention: Maintenance strategies in the treatment of addictive behaviors.* New York: Guilford.

Appendix A: Treatment Goals Assessment

Patient Name ________

File Number ________ Date ________

The following is a list of goals that people coming to treatment sometimes have. Please put an X in the box beside any of the goals that apply to you at the present. When you have done that, indicate in the next column any goal(s) that you think you need professional help to achieve.

	This is one of my present goals.	I need professional help to achieve this goal.
1. To deal with my problem of alcohol and/or drug use.	☐	☐
2. To learn to be less tense or anxious.	☐	☐

	This is one of my present goals.	I need professional help to achieve this goal.
3. To learn to stand up for my rights better, and to be able to express good or bad feelings directly.	☐	☐
4. To improve my relationship with members of my family (spouse, children, parents, etc.).	☐	☐
5. To be able to get along better socially.	☐	☐
6. To improve my ability to find and keep a job.	☐	☐
7. To learn to use my leisure time better.	☐	☐
8. To improve the nature of my living arrangements.	☐	☐
9. To deal effectively with legal problems that at present confront me.	☐	☐
10. To deal effectively with financial problems that at present confront me.	☐	☐
11. To increase my understanding of sexual problems and sexual behavior.	☐	☐

Summary

How many goals have you indicated? ________

Of the goals you indicated, which are the most important for you to solve at the moment?

My first most important goal is #________.
My second most important goals is #________.
My third most important goal is #________.
My fourth most important goal is #________.

Appendix B: Current Alcohol and Drug Use History

Patient Name ________

File Number ________ Date ________

Number of Days of Alcohol Use

Consumption per day	Past 30 Days	Past 31–60 Days	Past 61–90 Days
0 Drinks			
1-3 Standard Drinks			
4-6 Standard Drinks			
7+ Standard Drinks	*	*	*

*Average number of drinks on days where number of drinks is 7+.

	Primary Drugs	Pattern of Use: Daily	Daily/ Heavy Weekend	Weekend	Binges/ Runs	Occasional
1.						
2.						
3.						
4.						

Appendix C: Current Alcohol and Drug Use History (II)

Patient Name ________

File Number ________

Date ________

Drug class	Use Ever ✓=Yes X=No	Use in Past Year ✓=Yes X=No	Number of Days Used in Past 3 Months						Use a Current Prob. ✓=Yes X=No	Medical	Usual Mode of Admin. 1 Oral 2 Nasal 3 Inhale/ Smok'g 4 Inject 5 Other	Typical (Average) Dose
			Past 30 Days		Past 31–60 Days		Past 61–90 Days					
			Days of Use	Uses/ Day	Days of Use	Uses/ Day	Days of Use	Uses/ Days				
01 Alcohol			X	X	X	X	X	X	X	X	X	X
02 Cannabis									X	X		
03 Hallucinogens									X	X		
04 Narcotics												
05 Sed. Hypnotics												
06 Tranquilizers												
07 Cocaine									X	X		
08 Stimulants												
09 Solvents/Glue									X	X		
10 Other												

Appendix D: Lifestyle Scale

Patient Name ____________________________

File Number __________ Date __________

How well do you feel you are doing in each of these life areas? Mark the appropriate level with an X.

	Marital/ Family	Job/ School	Financial	Legal	Social relationships	Leisure	Physical health	Emotional health	Substance abuse	
Very Well										Very Well
Well										Well
So-So										So-So
Poorly										Poorly
Very Poorly										Very Poorly

Time 1 Intake/Clinical Assessment ☐

Time 2 Complete Interm Treatment ☐

Time 3 Complete Treatment ☐

Other, please specify ____________________________

Appendix E: Inventory of Drinking Situations—Short Form

Listed below are a number of situations or events in which some people drink heavily. Read each item carefully, and answer in terms of your own drinking over the past year.

If you "NEVER" drank heavily in that situation, circle "1."
If you "RARELY" drank heavily in that situation, circle "2."
If you "FREQUENTLY" drank heavily in that situation, circle "3."
If you "ALMOST ALWAYS" drank heavily in that situation, circle "4."

	I DRANK HEAVILY			
	Never	Rarely	Frequently	Almost always
1. When I had an argument with a friend.	1	2	3	4
2. When I felt uneasy in the presence of someone.	1	2	3	4

I DRANK HEAVILY	Never	Rarely	Frequently	Almost always
3. When someone criticized me.	1	2	3	4
4. When I would have trouble sleeping.	1	2	3	4
5. When I wanted to heighten my sexual enjoyment.	1	2	3	4
6. When other people around me made me tense.	1	2	3	4
7. When I would be out with friends and they would stop by a bar for a drink.	1	2	3	4
8. When I wanted to feel closer to someone I liked.	1	2	3	4
9. When I felt that I had let myself down.	1	2	3	4
10. When other people treated me unfairly.	1	2	3	4
11. When I would remember how good it tasted.	1	2	3	4
12. When I felt confident and relaxed.	1	2	3	4

	I DRANK HEAVILY			
	Never	Rarely	Frequently	Almost always
13. When I would convince myself that I was a new person now and could take a few drinks.	1	2	3	4
14. When I would pass by a liquor store.	1	2	3	4
15. When I felt drowsy and wanted to stay alert.	1	2	3	4
16. When I would be out with friends "on the town" and wanted to increase my enjoyment.	1	2	3	4
17. When I would unexpectedly find a bottle of my favorite booze.	1	2	3	4
18. When other people didn't seem to like me.	1	2	3	4
19. When I felt nauseous.	1	2	3	4
20. When I would wonder about my self-control over alcohol and would feel like having a drink to try it out.	1	2	3	4

	I DRANK HEAVILY			
	Never	Rarely	Frequently	Almost always
21. When other people interfered with my plans.	1	2	3	4
22. When everything was going well.	1	2	3	4
23. When I would be at a party and other people would be drinking.	1	2	3	4
24. When pressure would build up at work because of the demands of my supervisor.	1	2	3	4
25. When I was afraid that things weren't going to work out.	1	2	3	4
26. When I felt satisfied with something I had done.	1	2	3	4
27. When I would be in a restaurant and the people with me would order drinks.	1	2	3	4
28. When I wanted to celebrate with a friend.	1	2	3	4
29. When I was angry at the way things had turned out.	1	2	3	4

	I DRANK HEAVILY			
	Never	Rarely	Frequently	Almost always
30. When I would feel under a lot of pressure from family members at home.	1	2	3	4
31. When something good would happen and I would feel like celebrating.	1	2	3	4
32. When I would start to think that just one drink could cause no harm.	1	2	3	4
33. When I felt confused about what I should do.	1	2	3	4
34. When I would meet a friend and s/he would suggest that we have a drink together.	1	2	3	4
35. When I was not getting along well with others at work.	1	2	3	4
36. When I would be enjoying myself at a party and wanted to feel even better.	1	2	3	4
37. When I would suddenly have an urge to drink.	1	2	3	4

	I DRANK HEAVILY			
	Never	Rarely	Frequently	Almost always
38. When I wanted to prove to myself that I could take a few drinks without becoming drunk.	1	2	3	4
39. When there were fights at home.	1	2	3	4
40. When there were problems with people at work.	1	2	3	4
41. When I would be relaxed with a good friend and wanted to have a good time.	1	2	3	4
42. When my stomach felt like it was tied in knots.	1	2	3	4

The categorization of the 42 items into the eight categories of drinking situations is as follows: I. Intrapersonal Determinants: (1) Negative Emotional States—items #9, 25, 29, 33; (2) Negative Physical States—items #4, 15, 19, 42; (3) Positive Emotional States—items #12, 22, 26, 31; (4) Testing Personal Control—items #13, 20, 32, 38; and (5) Urges and Temptations—items #11, 14, 17, 37. II. Interpersonal Determinants: (1) Interpersonal Conflict, (a) Social Rejection—items #10, 18, 21; (b) Work Problems—items #24, 35, 40; (c) Tension—items #2, 3, 6; (d) Family Problems—items #1, 30, 39; (2) Social Pressure to Drink—items #7, 23, 27, 34; and (3) Positive Emotional States, (a) Social Drinking—items #16, 28, 36, 41; (b) Intimacy—items #5, 8.

Note: From H. M. Annis (1984). *Inventory of drinking situations* Addiction Research Foundation of Ontario. Ontario, Canada. © 1984. Reproduced by permission.

Appendix F: Situational Confidence Questionnaire

Listed below are a number of situations or events in which some people experience a drinking problem. Imagine yourself as you are right now in each of these situations. Indicate on the scale provided how confident you are that you would be able to resist the urge to drink heavily in that situation. Circle 100 if you are 100% confident right now that you could resist the urge to drink heavily; 80 if you are 80% confident; 60 if you are 60% confident. If you are more unconfident than confident, circle 40 to indicate that you are only 40% confident that you could resist the urge to drink heavily; 20 for 20% confident; 0 if you have no confidence at all about that situation.

	I WOULD BE ABLE TO RESIST THE URGE TO DRINK HEAVILY Not at all confident ... Very confident
1. If I had an argument with a friend.	0 20 40 60 80 100

	I WOULD BE ABLE TO RESIST THE URGE TO DRINK HEAVILY					
	Not at all confident					Very confident
2. If I felt uneasy in the presence of someone.	0	20	40	60	80	100
3. If someone criticized me.	0	20	40	60	80	100
4. If I would have trouble sleeping.	0	20	40	60	80	100
5. If I wanted to heighten my sexual enjoyment.	0	20	40	60	80	100
6. If other people around me made me tense.	0	20	40	60	80	100
7. If I would be out with friends and they would stop by a bar for a drink.	0	20	40	60	80	100
8. If I wanted to feel closer to someone I liked.	0	20	40	60	80	100
9. If I felt that I had let myself down.	0	20	40	60	80	100
10. If other perople treated me unfairly.	0	20	40	60	80	100
11. If I would remember how good it tasted.	0	20	40	60	80	100
12. If I felt confident and relaxed.	0	20	40	60	80	100
13. If I would convince myself that I was a new person now and could take a few drinks.	0	20	40	60	80	100
14. If I would pass by a liquor store.	0	20	40	60	80	100

	I WOULD BE ABLE TO RESIST THE URGE TO DRINK HEAVILY					
	Not at all confident					Very confident
15. If I felt drowsy and wanted to stay alert.	0	20	40	60	80	100
16. If I would be out with friends "on the town" and wanted to increase my enjoyment.	0	20	40	60	80	100
17. If I would unexpectedly find a bottle of my favorite booze.	0	20	40	60	80	100
18. If other people didn't seem to like me.	0	20	40	60	80	100
19. If I felt nauseous.	0	20	40	60	80	100
20. If I would wonder about my self-control over alcohol and would feel like having a drink to try it out.	0	20	40	60	80	100
21. If other people interfered with my plans.	0	20	40	60	80	100
22. If everything was going well.	0	20	40	60	80	100
23. If I would be at a party and other people would be drinking.	0	20	40	60	80	100
24. If pressure would build up at work because of the demands of my supervisor.	0	20	40	60	80	100
25. If I were afraid that things weren't going to work out.	0	20	40	60	80	100
26. If I felt satisfied with something I had done.	0	20	40	60	80	100

	I WOULD BE ABLE TO RESIST THE URGE TO DRINK HEAVILY					
	Not at all confident					Very confident
27. If I would be in a restaurant and the people with me would order drinks.	0	20	40	60	80	100
28. If I wanted to celebrate with a friend.	0	20	40	60	80	100
29. If I were angry at the way things had turned out.	0	20	40	60	80	100
30. If I would feel under a lot of pressure from family members at home.	0	20	40	60	80	100
31. If something good would happen and I would feel like celebrating.	0	20	40	60	80	100
32. If I would start to think that just one drink could cause no harm.	0	20	40	60	80	100
33. If I felt confused about what I should do.	0	20	40	60	80	100
34. If I would meet a friend and s/he would suggest that we have a drink together.	0	20	40	60	80	100
35. If I were not getting along well with others at work.	0	20	40	60	80	100
36. If I would be enjoying myself at a party and wanted to feel even better.	0	20	40	60	80	100
37. If I would suddenly have an urge to drink.	0	20	40	60	80	100

	I WOULD BE ABLE TO RESIST THE URGE TO DRINK HEAVILY					
	Not at all confident					Very confident
38. If I wanted to prove to myself that I could take a few drinks without becoming drunk.	0	20	40	60	80	100
39. If there were fights at home.	0	20	40	60	80	100
40. If there were problems with people at work.	0	20	40	60	80	100
41. If I would be relaxed with a good friend and wanted to have a good time.	0	20	40	60	80	100
42. If my stomach felt like it was tied in knots.	0	20	40	60	80	100

12

Response to Chemical Impairment: Policy and Program Initiatives

Tonda L. Hughes and Ann Solari-Twadell

Nursing practice in the United States is monitored by agencies which regulate the licensing of professionals and by professional nursing organizations that promulgate ethical and professional standards.

When a nurse develops a drug problem or becomes addicted, the likelihood that the nurse's professional performance will be adversely affected is great. The risk of harm caused by nurses whose skills and judgement are impaired is a concern that must be addressed at the professional, institutional, and individual levels.

Legal Requirements

All nurses in the United States must be licensed, and although the regulations and requirements vary among the states, the primary purpose is to ensure safe, competent nursing practice.

Actions relating to nurse impairment taken by regulatory boards or committees generally fall into one of three categories: (1) action involving drugs; (2) action involving administration of medications; and (3) misconduct related to nursing practice. Impairment caused by chemical dependency most frequently falls into the first category. From 1980 to 1984 state boards of nursing reported disciplinary hearings for 2,364 registered nurses and 1,128 licensed practical nurses involving violations of the nurse practice act within this category (Gerace, 1985).

Requirements for reporting and actions taken against nurses' licenses vary from state to state. Many states have mandatory reporting or "snitch" laws. And, while some states may deal more leniently with nurses whose impairment has not obviously infringed upon the welfare of clients/patients or the employing institution, in all states stealing or diverting narcotics is a felony, and reporting to federal law enforcement agencies is required.

In 1985 the National Nurses Society on Addiction (NNSA) developed a "Statement on Model Diversion Legislation for Chemically Impaired Nurses" (see Appendix to this chapter). NNSA supports the use of alternative or "diversion" programming for nurses by all states. The model statement consists of language, content, and format that can be adapted for use by individual states. Diversion programs are voluntary, nonpunitive alternatives to disciplinary action that provide help for the nurse while ensuring that patient care is not affected by drug abuse or addiction. Such programs remove the nurse from practice during the active phase of addiction and continue to monitor practice during a designated period of recovery. A few states have already implemented (or are working to develop) programs through which nurses may obtain treatment without being reported, or at least with less long-term risk to their careers.

In states that do not have alternative programs, mandatory reporting laws are viewed primarily as punitive and have not proved effective in regulating practice. Nurses are reluctant to report colleagues when disclosure will almost certainly lead to loss of employment, loss of license, or both. This reluctance deters early intervention and prolongs risk of harm to both the addicted nurse and the client or patient.

Professional Response

A profession has both a responsibility to its members and an obligation to preserve public safety. These responsibilities were addressed in 1982 when the American Nurses Association adopted a resolution "to address health problems that compromise nurses' ability to function within the standards and code of conduct for professional practice" (ANA, 1984). The resolution called for the development of guidelines for assistance programs, the encouragement of nurses' employers to offer appropriate services *prior* to disciplinary action, and the establishment of mechanisms to collect and disseminate information related to the problem of impairment among nurses (ANA, 1982). This resolution evolved from the work of the Task Force on Addictions and Psychological Dysfunctions. This group is comprised of representatives from several professional organizations including the American Nurses' Association (ANA), the National Nurses Society on Addiction (NNSA), and the Drug and Alcohol Nurses Association (DANA).

Nursing specialty organizations such as NNSA and DANA have been particularly active in working to ameliorate the problem of chemical dependency among nurses. For example, a committee of the NNSA has been involved for several years in gathering and disseminating information about the issue of professional impairment. Most recently, the committee conducted a national survey of impaired nurse programs. The resulting document provides up-to-date information about programming for chemically impaired nurses in the individual states (see appendix).

Currently, approximately 28 state nurses' associations have peer assistance programs in place, and an additional 20 states have formed committees or are in the process of developing some form of peer assistance program (Green, 1987; Naegle, 1988). State programs vary significantly in focus and level of activity. For example, some state programs provide only education and referral. In Florida, California, New Mexico, Texas, and New York nursing groups have successfully lobbied for statutes that allow chemically impaired nurses who voluntarily enter treatment to avoid the usual disciplinary procedures. The Louisiana State Nurses' Association has established a similar, though less formal alternative to disciplinary action via a memorandum of understanding with the board of nursing. Such provisions recognize that addiction is an illness and assume that a rehabilitative rather than a punitive approach is more effective in dealing with the problem.

Whatever the activities of the state programs, the goal of each is to assist nurses suffering from addiction (or psychological dysfunction), while ensuring that professional standards are maintained. Thus, the recent proliferation of programs among the states is encouraging. However, the continuation of activities initiated by nurses involved in these programs depends on the development of policies supportive of the aims of the programs, as well as the procurement of resources to finance such programs.

Institutional Response

Just as the profession is responsible for setting standards of practice, individual institutions set performance expectations through the development of policies and procedures, quality assurance guidelines, and performance evaluation criteria. Such standards are effective only when they are explicitly stated and communicated to all levels of nursing staff. Clear standards of performance facilitate early identification of problems. Documentation of substandard performance is recognized as key in identifying nurses who are abusing alcohol or drugs or who are chemically dependent.

Progressive activity at the institutional level has lagged behind that occurring at the state level. Although chemical dependency is now recognized as affecting significant numbers of nurses, few hospitals or other health care institutions have policies for dealing with the problem. A recent survey of top-level nursing administrators from acute care hospitals in one midwestern state found that only 39% of the hospitals surveyed have written policies related to nurses who abuse substances or are chemically dependent (Hughes, 1988).

The absence of institutional policies and/or guidelines acts as a fundamental barrier to intervention and, as such, allows the chemically-dependent nurse to become progressively sicker, places the clients or patients at increased risk of harm, and exposes the employer/institution to greater risk of liability. In contrast, policies such as the Fitness-for-Duty policy described in Chapter 10 benefit all involved.

In addition to policies that guide response when chemical dependency is suspected or confirmed, policies should be developed that focus on reentry following treatment. While concerns understandably exist regarding the hiring or rehiring of a recovering chemically dependent nurse, the benefits of doing so are increasingly being recognized and reported (Abbott, 1987; Catanzarite, 1987; Sullivan, 1986).

An effective return-to-work policy should not only spell out how the recovering nurse will be monitored, but must also address the issue of relapse. Chemical dependency is a chronic, progressing, and sometimes recurring health problem; relapse must be recognized as a potential hazard. Policies that do not address relapse, or require immediate termination in cases of relapse deny that it may take more than one attempt to maintain abstinence. Such stipulations will ultimately erode the supportive spirit of the policy. A more effective policy outlines in detail what is to happen in the case of relapse so that nurses in trouble are quickly identified and offered the needed help to restore health and professional functioning.

Finally, to help chemically dependent nurses quickly and effectively, the reporting nurse must not fear legal reprisal for wrongful accusation. Nurses fear that if they take action either by reporting or intervening in a situation where chemical dependency is suspected but not confirmed, they may be held legally liable for defamation. Chaney (1987) discusses the importance of "safe harbor" statutes that provide immunity to supervisors or colleagues who report to the state licensing board nurses suspected of being chemically dependent. Similarly, communication between staff and supervisors, is considered privileged if restricted to co-workers, supervisors or others who are in a position to be legally affected (p. 63). However, as mentioned earlier, nurses may still be reluctant to report colleagues who are chemically dependent when it is likely that such disclosures will result in termination, loss of license, or both.

Policy Implementation

The importance of policies and standards concerning chemical impairment among nurses has been increasingly recognized and reported (Abbott, 1987; ANA, 1984; Barr & Lerner, 1984; Chaney, 1987; Gerace, 1985; Hughes, 1986).

Although the effectiveness of policy in altering behavior is not well documented, a number of factors have been identified that are believed to influence a policy's impact.

One factor, termed "diffusion" (Gray, 1977; Walker, 1969), involves the extent to which a new policy or innovation spreads from one institution or state to another institution or state. Diffusion is the process by which the communication of an idea (or policy) over time leads to the adoption of the idea or policy by a new group. As institutions, nursing associations, and state legislatures adopt policies on professional impairment, the communication of the fact will have an impact on policy development in other institutions and states. By necessity, administrators or state officials view the policy adopted in other institutions or states as a standard or point of departure from which to formulate their own standards. In nursing, this process is beginning to occur, as legislative changes and alternative methods of disciplining chemically dependent nurses are instituted in various states. Professional involvement in these activities is essential to initiate standards that will effectively guide institutions and individual practitioners in dealing with the problem of impaired practice. As policies that serve the interests of both the public and the chemically impaired nurse are adopted and implemented, such actions will begin to "diffuse" into other locations. Diffusion is also occurring through the efforts of various professional organizations to disseminate information about chemical impairment.

Other important factors influencing the success or failure of policy implementation have been discussed by Brewer and deLeon (1983). These factors include (1) source of the policy, (2) clarity of the policy, (3) support for the policy, (4) complexity of administration, (5) incentives for implementors, and (6) resource allocation.

While the same factors are important in influencing policy on an institutional level as well, a recent legislative bill developed in Illinois exemplifies the significance of the above factors on the success or failure of policy on the state level. The bill was introduced by an Illinois senator following heightened, and rather sensationalized, publicity, in Illinois and nationally about drug use and addiction among nurses. In its original form, the bill did not emanate from or have the support of nurses. The bill was opposed by the Illinois Nurses' Association, who disagreed with its original intent, which severely restricted the options of both chemically impaired nurses and those responsible for dealing with impaired nursing practice. That intent was modified through the work of nurses from the Illinois Nurses' Association (INA) and the Illinois Peer Assistance Network for Nurses (PANN), who convinced the senator that the bill in its original form would draw tremendous opposition from the nursing constituency, and more importantly, that it would not be helpful in rehabilitating chemically impaired nurses.

A revised form of the bill was passed as an amendment to the Illinois Nursing Act. Essentially, the bill stated that nursing administrators are required to report to the state licensing board any nurse suspected of being chemically impaired. The amendment included a clause stating that the administrator may choose not to file the report if the nurse completes a program of treatment and is monitored by the administrator or employing institution.

The impact of the bill was questionable from the beginning because of the "vagaries" included, and because nursing administrators as a group interpreted the amendment as limiting their actions, rather than broadening them. Thus, they had no incentive to comply with either the spirit or the letter of this law. Furthermore, there were few tangible incentives to encourage nursing administrators to adhere to the tenets of the amendment. For example, the bill carried no penalty for failure to act according to its mandate. As a result, an additional amendment, initiated by the Illinois Hospital Association via the Illinois Organization of Nurse Executives, has been added. While this amendment was intended to clarify nurse administrators' responsibilities, and thus strengthen the intent of the bill, its effectiveness remains uncertain. Similar difficulties have been identified in other states and it appears likely that failure to comply is typical in many states that have mandatory reporting laws.

As is often the case, the Illinois legislation was not initiated by nurses. Even though nursing groups were able to rally enough support to force some revisions, the resulting compromise bill has not been an effective response to the problem. The fact that nursing administrators continue to have some difficulty interpreting and thus implementing the law illustrates the importance of active participation of nurses in the development of policies and standards that guide professional practice.

Summary and Conclusion

A general lack of understanding of addiction, coupled with a lack of financial resources, serves as a formidable barrier to more effective policies and standards on the problem of impaired practice. The cost of developing, publicizing, and lobbying a bill is significant. Implementation of alternative programming for nurses such as those instituted in California and Florida require considerable resources. However, it is becoming increasingly apparent that the volunteer efforts that have heretofore initiated and maintained most state-level peer assistance programs cannot be sustained indefinitely. The nursing profession and individual nurses must be willing to work toward and support more enduring alternative plans. An example of one such means of support being proposed in a number of states is an increase in licensure fees to cover or offset the costs of assistance programs.

Self regulation and monitoring of nursing practice to ensure that high standards of professional performance are maintained is considered the hallmark of a true profession (Donabedian, 1976). To maintain high standards of professional practice, nursing must monitor its members. The responsibilities of nurses to the consumer and to each other have been articulated by the American Nurses' Association Code for Nurses. This code states that the nurse will act to safeguard the client and the public when health care is affected by incompetent, unethical, or illegal practice (ANA, 1976).

By necessity, such standards touch directly upon issues of impaired practice. For example, the decision-making process necessary to address issues of impaired practice must be a systematic, thoughtful one, for the ethical and professional dilemmas confronting the nursing profession in regard to this problem have no easy solutions. In deciding to act, the individual nurse in any position must consider (1) personal beliefs and attitudes, (2) professional ethics, (3) professional standards, (4) values of the employing organization or institution, and (5) legal requirements of state licensing boards and regulatory agencies (Naegle, 1985). Currently, because of the general lack of knowledge among nurses and administrators about chemical dependency as well as the absence of guidelines for action, the decision to act is too often an arbitrary one that does little to assist the impaired nurse to obtain much needed help.

At a broader level, nurses must be aware of the effects legislation and policy have on the profession as a whole. Every nurse has the responsibility to understand not only the implications of policy on practice, but also the effects of addiction on safe practice and the general welfare of the profession. Activities at both local and national levels must continue to be supported, for they are essential if primary responsibility for practice is to be maintained within the profession.

Institutional standards in the form of policy are important as guidelines for action for nursing administrators and other nursing staff who are confronted with the problem of impaired functioning among employees and peers. Such standards help to ensure equitable and beneficial responses to nurses who experience impaired functioning because of drug or alcohol use. Until institutional policies are the norm, legislative policies that include provisions for assisting the chemically impaired nurse into treatment and for supporting reentry following treatment must be developed and promoted. Conversely, legislative policies, especially if nurses are involved in their development, can provide an official and uniform standard for the development of policies at the institutional level. This is particularly important when issues that evoke strong feelings and opinions are involved.

Once developed, such policies provide a framework for future action, including the development of educational and research activities, which are essential if the problem of impairment among nurses is to be treated effectively, humanely, and professionally.

References

Abbott, C. A. (1987). The impaired nurse. Part III: Management Strategies. *AORN Journal, 46*(6), 1104–1115.

American Nurses' Association. (1976). *Code for nurses with interpretive statements.* Kansas City: Author.

American Nurses' Association House of Delegates. (1982). *Action on alcohol and drug misuse and psychological dysfunctions among nurses.* Resolution 5, adopted June 29, 1982.

American Nurses' Association. (1984). *Addictions and psychological dysfunctions in nursing: The profession's response to the problem.* Kansas City: Author.

Barr, M. A., & Lerner, W.D. (1984). The impaired nurse: A management issue. *Nursing Economics, 2,* 196–201.

Brewer, G. D., & deLeon, P. (1983). *The foundations of policy analysis.* Homewood, Illinois: The Dorsey Press.

Chaney, E. A. (1987). Nurses and chemical dependency: policy considerations. *Journal of Pediatric Nursing* 2(1), 61–63.

Catanzarite, A. (1987, March). *Florida's alternative program: A win/win situation.* Presented at the Fifth National Impaired Nurse Symposium and Research Conference: Programming—What Works and What Doesn't. Emory University and National Nurses Society on Addictions, Atlanta.

Donabedian, A. (1976). Forward. In *The nursing audit and self recognition in nursing practice (2nd ed.).* New York: Appleton Century Crofts.

Gerace, L. (1985, August). *Analysis of policy and program implementation for the impaired nurse: what is being done in the United States.* Proceedings of the 34th International Congress on Alcoholism and Drug Dependence, 2, (pp. 53–55.). Calgary, AB.

Gray, V. (1977). Innovations in the states: A diffusion study. *American Political Science Review, 63*(9), 880–899.

Green, P. L. (1987, March). *Programming for Impaired Nurses.* Presented at the Fifth national Impaired Nurse Symposium and Research Conference. Emory University and National Nurses Society on Addictions, Atlanta.

Hughes, T. L. (1986, June). *Chemical impairment in nursing: Policy and program implementation.* Presented at the 32nd International Institute on the Prevention and Treatment of Alcoholism, Budapest, Hungary.

Hughes, T. L. (1988, March). *Chief nurse executives' responses to chemically dependent nurses: The influence of institutional, personal, and contextual factors.* Presented at the Sixth National Impaired Nurse Symposium and Research Conference: Legal, Moral & Ethical Issues, Atlanta.

Naegle, M. A. (1985). Creative management of impaired nursing practice. *Nursing Administration Quarterly,* 9(3), 16–26.

Naegle, M. A. (1988, March). *The state of the art and ethical issues: Where we are now.* Presented at the Sixth National Impaired Nurse Symposium and Research Conference: Legal, Moral & Ethical Issues, Atlanta.

Sullivan, E. (1986). Cost savings of retaining chemically dependent nurses. *Nursing Economics,* 4(4), 196–199.

Walker, J. L. (1969). The diffusion of innovations among American states. *American Political Science Review, 63*(9), 880–899.

Appendix: Statement on Model Diversion Legislation for Chemically Impaired Nurses of the National Nurses Society on Addictions (NNSA)

Over recent years, state nurses associations, specialty nursing groups and others, have worked to develop positions, mechanisms and peer assistance programs to help impaired nurses. Their goal(s) have been to assist nurses, whose practice is either actually or potentially affected, to find appropriate treatment for their illness, thus assisting and protecting both nurse and patient.

The nurse suffering from the primary illness of alcohol and/or drug addiction has long been a concern, not just of the profession, but also of state regulatory bodies. State nursing boards have as their primary function, the protection of the public. In fulfilling that responsibility, they have often been in the position of being required to discipline a nurse for an act of commission or omission resulting purely from what is acknowledged to be the nurse's illness. Few boards have been pleased with this requirement, but have not felt that alternatives were available to them.

The National Nurses Society on Addictions, after observing the legislative efforts of such states as Florida, California and Hawaii, the programs developed by other professions, and the handling of other violations requiring due process, believes that a model diversion program for nurses, to be adopted by each state, could be of great assistance to the Boards of Nursing, individual nurses, our profession and our patients.

The following is a model statement and diversion legislation that NNSA hopes will be helpful in dealing with this issue in a safe, effective and humane manner.

Model Statement

The ____________________ State Board of Nursing, in the matter of nurses whose functioning is impaired by alcoholism or drug addiction, recognizes:

1. that alcoholism and drug addiction are primary illnesses and should be treated as such.
2. that problems resulting from these illnesses can include personal, legal and health problems that may impair the nurse's personal health and ability to practice safely.
3. that nurses who develop these illnesses can, with appropriate treatment, be helped to recover.
4. that programs of assistance that include treatment and monitoring, as an alternative to a disciplinary process, have been particularly effective in rehabilitating the professional and in protecting the public.
5. that nurses who are willing to cooperate with a program of assistance to them and accept treatment for these illnesses should be allowed to avoid disciplinary action provided they cooperate fully with recommended treatment and comply with the requirements for monitoring of their continued well being after formal treatment is completed.

Therefore, the ____________________ State Board of Nursing supports the enactment of an amendment to the nurse practice act in this state calling for a diversion procedure for nurses who have been (or are likely to be) charged with violating the nurse practice act, but who are willing to stipulate to certain facts and enter a program approved by the Board.

Diversion Procedure

Section ___________________.

It is the intent of the Legislature that the Board of Nursing (hereafter referred to as the Board) seek ways and means to identify and rehabilitate nurses whose competency may be impaired due to abuse of drugs or alcohol, so that such nurses can be treated and can return to or continue the practice of nursing in a manner which will benefit the public. It is further the intent of the Legislature that the Board of Nursing, by implementing this legislation, will establish a diversion procedure as a voluntary alternative to traditional disciplinary actions and as an alternative to lengthy and costly investigations and administrative proceedings against such nurses but also having adequate safeguards for the patient.

Section ___________________.

As used in this statute:

1. "Program" means a formal, structured regimen, sponsored by a recognized group, designed to and capable of assisting addicted nurses and referring them for evaluation and treatment, including mutual help groups and monitoring them for a period of at least two years.
   a. "Peer Assistance Program" means a program administered by professional nurses for the purpose of assisting their colleagues in obtaining evaluation, treatment, monitoring and on-going support for the purpose of arresting their addiction.
   b. "Employee Assistance Program" means a program offered by an employer of nurses for the purpose of identifying and assisting them in obtaining evaluation, treatment, monitoring and on-going support for the purpose of arresting their addiction.

   c. "Approved Program" means either a Peer Assistance Program or an Employee Assistance Program that has been approved and accepted by the Board of Nursing as having the ability to meet the requirements of this act by referring nurses for evaluation and treatment and by providing ongoing support and monitoring for those nurses.
2. "Treatment" refers to a formalized plan carried out by a chemical dependency professional in either an in-patient or out-patient setting, designed to provide primary care, leading to rehabilitation.
3. "Committee" refers to a Diversion Evaluation Committee appointed by the Board to carry out such duties as are herein described.

Section____________________.

The Board shall appoint one or more Diversion Evaluation Committees.

1. The committee will be composed of five persons:
   a. two registered nurses and one licensed practical nurse, all licensed under this chapter. The Board will give consideration to recommendations of nursing organizations and shall give priority consideration to the appointment of nurses who have recovered from impairment or who specialize in addictions nursing.
   b. two members not necessarily licensed as nurses but who have experience or knowledge in the evaluation or management of persons impaired by chemical dependency.
2. Each appointment shall be at the pleasure of the Board for a term not to exceed four years. The Board, at its discretion, may stagger the terms of the initial members appointed. A member may be reappointed once.
3. The members of the Committee will serve without pay, but will be reimbursed for the expenses incurred in the discharge of their duties at a rate determined by the state for all state business.
4. The Committee shall elect a chairperson and a vice-chairperson.
5. The Committee will review the request of each nurse for diver-

sion, according to criteria established by the Board, and recommend to the Board either in favor or against diversion. In all cases where the Committee has recommended diversion the Board shall grant diversion, except that for good cause shown the Board may disregard the Committee's recommendation and deny diversion.

6. The Committee will review the regimen developed by a Program for each nurse and will determine whether that nurse may safely continue or resume the practice of nursing while on diversion.
7. The Committee will hear reports from the nurses on diversion and from the Programs as to each nurse's progress and cooperation and will, in turn, report and refer to the Board all relevant information and requests for action according to guidelines established by the Board.

Section ____________________.

One or more programs may be designated and contracted with as approved programs by the Board to carry out this article. Such programs must meet the following requirements:

1. Peer Assistance Programs will be designated for approval by the Board after consideration of the recommendation of the Committee and providing:
   a. They are sponsored by or in conjunction with the state nurses' association.
   b. that staff and/or volunteers of the program are educated, experienced, and supervised, appropriate to the level of involvement in the program.
   c. they include within their program, referral to bona fide chemical dependency treatment centers, e.g., those accredited by the Joint Commission of the Accreditation of Hospitals or those licensed by the state as such.
   d. they refer to mutual help groups, e.g., Alcoholics Anonymous, Narcotics Anonymous.
   e. they monitor participants for a period of two years including the random examination of body fluids as appropriate.
   f. they agree to immediately report to the Committee, any nurse that does not cooperate and comply with the requirements of the program.

   g. they agree to report to the Committee, regularly and when requested, the status of individual nurses as to cooperation and progress, including the overall status of the Program.
2. Employee Assistance Programs will be designated Programs for approval by the Board after consideration of the recommendations of the Committee providing:
   a. they have staff that have had a minimum of two years experience in the addictions field and in a health care agency or are directly supervised by someone with such experience.
   b. they include within their program, referral to bona fide treatment centers, e.g., those accredited by the Joint Commission on the Accreditation of Hospitals or licensed by the state as such.
   c. they refer to mutual help groups, e.g., Alcoholics Anonymous, Narcotics Anonymous.
   d. they monitor participants for a period of two years including the use of random drug screens.
   e. they agree to immediately report to the Committee any nurse that does not cooperate and comply with the requirements of the Program.
   f. they agree to report to the Committee, regularly and when requested, the status of individual nurses as to cooperation and progress and the overall status of the Program.

If no suitable programs are available in the state, the Board may contract for the development of such a program, providing it has no direct control over the program.

Section ____________________.

The Board may increase the licensing fee for each nurse in the state, not to exceed $5, to cover the cost of implementation and maintenance of this article.

Section ____________________.

Any nurse, appearing before the Board for a violation of the nurse practice act due to an apparent addiction to alcohol or other drugs will be advised of the opportunity for diversion. The nurse will be advised of the procedure to be followed and to be eligible, such nurse must stipulate to certain facts, waive a speedy hearing or trial and become a participant in, and agree to cooperate with, an approved program. The Board may grant diversion to a nurse after reviewing the nurse's application for diversion and the recommendation of the Committee. Subsequent failure to cooperate and comply shall be reported to the Board by the Committee and may result in termination of the diversion procedure.

Section ___________________.

The Board of Nursing will develop a written diversion agreement which sets forth the requirements which must be met by the nurse and the conditions under which the diversion procedure may be successfully completed or terminated due to lack of cooperation or compliance. Time already spent in an approved program may be taken into consideration by the Board in determining the length of diversion.

Section ___________________.

Records of the approved programs and treatment as they pertain to the diversion procedure shall be kept confidential, with the exception of the reporting as to whether or not the nurse is cooperating and complying, and are not subject to discovery or subpoena.

Section ___________________.

During the time the nurse is on diversion he or she will be required to remain in an approved program. Participation in a satisfactory program in another state may be approved upon application and a showing of need. The diversionee may not practice in another state without the knowledge of the Board of that state of his/her participation in the diversion program.

Section ___________________.

After a period of five years, provided no additional occurrences of alcohol or drug related violations or crimes have occurred, the records of the diversion and charges will be purged upon request of the nurse.

Section ___________________.

Any person making reports to the Board or to the Committee regarding a nurse suspected of practicing while impaired or reports of a nurse's progress or lack of progress in a Program shall be immune from civil action for defamation or other cause of action resulting from such reports, provided that such report is made in good faith and with some reasonable basis in fact.

Section ____________________.

The Board of Nursing, any Committee or member thereof appointed by the Board, any Program or its staff or volunteers, any Treatment agency or its staff or volunteers, or any nurse, licensed to practice under the laws of this State that has supervisory responsibility over the practice of nursing by a diversionee, or an employer of such a diversionee, shall not be liable for any civil damages resulting from the diversionee's negligence in his/her practice, or the fact that such diversionee's license to practice was not revoked, or that such diversionee was employed or retained in employment except for such damages which may result from such person, Board or group's negligence or wanton acts or omissions in the supervision of the impaired nurse.

CAUTION

Mandatory reporting is not included in this model. This is a difficult issue and is felt to be, in general, counter-productive. Should it be in force in certain states or considered for inclusion with this proposed legislation, an exemption should be allowed for those nurses working in treatment programs or programs of assistance.

We suggest that close attention be paid to the section on the funding of the act. It should be clear that the Board can use that money to pay for the cost of programs when needed.

Persons not familiar with the legislative process should be warned that the passage of the act is not the final action. The drafting of the rules and regulations and guidelines that implement the act are also important and will require the attention of interested persons.

National Nurses Society on Addictions, 2506 Gross Point Road, Evanston, IL 60201, (312) 475-7300.

13

Future Directions in Research and Prevention

Mary R. Haack

In recent years, increasing attention has been devoted to the problem of impaired functioning among practicing nurses. Impaired functioning results from the presence of certain dysfunctions related to alcohol and drug misuse or psychological problems that interfere with the professional's judgment and the delivery of safe, high-quality care (ANA, 1984). As a result, many articles, conferences, programs, and policies have been generated on the topic. The purpose of this chapter is to provide an overview of the research on the nurse whose functioning is impaired, and by so doing, attempt to give an accurate picture of what we know and what we do not know about impairment and its prevention.

Reports of problems stemming from alcohol, drug use, and psychological dysfunctions among nurses are not new. Nightingale's correspondence contains references to nurses who had to be dismissed for drunkenness. In general, nursing care was provided by convicts, prostitutes, and alcoholics during the Nightingale period. The exceptions occurred in countries where religious sisters provided care for the sick. Nursing reform and the establishment of training schools based on Nightingale's system marked the beginning of modern nursing as we know it today. Nightingale's initiative not only attempted to overcome the knowledge and skill deficits within nursing, but also to improve the image of nursing. To do this, Nightingale promoted the idea that nurses were called to a quasi-religious vocation; caring for the sick was doing God's work. To guide this work, numerous books on nursing ethics and etiquette were written. The ideas expressed in this literature reflect the moralistic attitudes toward substance addiction prevalent during that time in England and the United States. Although the Nightingale reforms successfully promoted professionalism within nursing, they also contributed to the denial of the nurse's humanity and to the lack of action by the profession toward members whose practice was impaired.

While even today the profession does not fully accept its responsibility for the problem of impairment among nurses, the media has made the problem impossible to ignore. It is not uncommon for various aspects of impairment to be dramatized on prime-time television and in the movies. The image of a handcuffed nurse being led from a place of employment by a law enforcement officer has appeared in newspapers, magazines, and television news reports across the country.

As a result of this recent focus on the problem of impairment within nursing, extreme statements regarding the magnitude of the problem have been made in the popular press and within nursing circles. While sensational statistics may aid in the promotion and development of programs for nurses who are suffering from addiction, exaggerating the problem is no more helpful than to moralize against it in the Nightingale tradition. Only when we understand the nature and the scope of the problem can we effectively intervene and prevent the suffering that drug addiction, alcoholism, and psychological dysfunction can cause.

The research reviewed in this chapter was identified through a search of the data banks from the National Clearinghouse on Alcohol and Drug Information (NCADI) and Nursing & Allied Health (CINAHL). Sources of information include surveys, clinical observations, anecdotes, the popular press, and gossip. For the purpose of this chapter, the studies have been divided into the following categories: epidemiologic studies, social/psychological studies, intervention/evaluation studies, policy studies, prevention studies, and investigations that explore theoretical models.

Epidemiologic Studies

Mortality

Mortality rate is defined as the number of deaths from a given disease. Alcohol- and drug-related mortality statistics are usually related to motor vehicle accidents, liver disease, and violent deaths (homicide and suicide) reported on death certificates. It is now popular in the United States to state that one nurse dies each day as a result of an addictive disease, but there are, in fact, no data to support this statistic (Television movie by Riche, Rudnick, Epstein, & Anstaugh, 1986). The Bay Area Task Force in San Francisco examined death certificates of nurses in the city and county of San Francisco for a six-month period in 1983 and found that 39 nurses died as a result of alcoholism or drug dependency. The average age of these nurses was 31. It was concluded from this study that one nurse dies every five weeks as a result of an addictive disorder (Buxton, Jessup, & Landry, 1985).

Although there have been studies on the leading causes of death in nurses, this information has not been published in the nursing literature. A study on female mortality by occupation in the state of California between the years of 1979 and 1981 revealed suicide to be the leading cause of death in nurses (State of California, 1987). This finding is consistent with similar studies in Wisconsin (Katz, 1983), Washington (Milham, 1983), and Great Britain (Reg. Gen., 1978). The relationship of these suicides to specific psychiatric disorders is not known. Certainly this finding is alarming and warrants further investigation. Although one could quickly jump to the conclusion that these deaths are substance-abuse related, we do not have the data to support that hypothesis. It would be a significant contribution to the literature if a nurse researcher would do a systematic postmortem investigation of these deaths.

In general, women make more suicide attempts than men, and those with a medical or nursing background are more in danger of succeeding because they are more knowledgeable about effective methods. Bissell and Haberman (1984) report that 31% of their sample of addicted nurses reported suicide attempts. These data are important but cannot be generalized beyond the samples studied. Other studies examining death certificates must be done to produce an accurate picture of mortality related to substance abuse and depressive disorders among nurses. Only then can the data be generalized to the total nursing population.

Morbidity

Morbidity is the statistic that establishes the incidence and prevalence of an illness within a population. Most often this number is derived from discharge data from community hospitals, treatment programs, and emergency rooms. Manifestations of alcohol and drug morbidity are determined by diagnosis of cirrhosis, psychosis, and dependent and nondependent abuse of substances. An investigation of alcohol and drug morbidity rates has never been done for nurses. Nevertheless, it has been stated on national television that there are 200,000 addicted nurses in the U.S. (Riche, Rudnick, Epstein, & Anstaugh, 1986). The source for this statistic is not known. Since there are now approximately two million nurses in the United States and popular belief has it that nurses are at greater risk for the development of an addiction, it is possible that this number is derived by doubling the 5% expected rate of alcoholism in women in the general population. This projection is merely a guess with no data to support it.

The statistics we do have are based on the number of drug-related cases heard before a state licensing board and the number of license revocations that have resulted from a substance abuse problem. The American Nurses Association (1984) reports that 68% of all state board actions over a 12-month period stemmed from impaired functioning related to substance dependence. This statistic establishes that chemical dependency is indeed a serious problem within the profession; however, it does not establish the number of cases of alcoholism or drug addiction in existence at a given time in a specific geographical area or the number of new cases occurring within a specific time frame. This work still needs to be done.

Population Studies

Since alcohol and drugs are such significant factors in impairment, it is important to determine if nurses are more at risk for addiction to these substances than is the general population. Three investigators have done preliminary studies designed to answer this question.

Billings (1986) studied a random sample of nurses in North Carolina and found that they drink less than other women in the general population. Haack and Harford (1984, 1985) studied patterns of alcohol and drug use among nursing students in an American university and found that their alcohol use was comparable to other college students, but that their drug use was less. Similarly, McAuliffe and colleagues (1984) have investigated a small sample of nursing students in connection with their study on medical students and found that they do not differ from other college women in their use of alcohol or drugs.

Engs (1982) reported that the drinking pattern of Australian nursing students was similar to that of other students, but that they had greater access to drugs. An investigation of Nigerian nursing students revealed less alcohol use but more analgesic, amphetamine, and tranquilizer use when compared with United States nursing students (Haack & Harford, 1987). It is important to note that the per capita consumption of alcohol is significantly lower in Nigeria than in the United States because of the greater number of Moslems in the population and the public policies controlling distribution of alcohol and other recreational drugs (Addiction Research Foundation, 1984). These studies are only representative of the samples investigated. None of these investigations can be generalized to all nursing students or to all nurses. To date, no research accurately assesses the incidence and prevalence of alcohol and drug dependence within the nursing profession as a whole. It is also important to note that none of the investigations done so far support the belief that nurses have a greater prevalence of substance use than the general population.

Social/Psychological Studies

Risk Factors

Clinical Specialty Area

Most of the nursing addiction literature focuses on specialties that have greater access to controlled substances, such as nurses who work in anesthesiology, orthopedics, or critical care (Norris, 1986).

However, since there are no data on the incidence and prevalence of abuse and dependence, there is no way to identify accurately who within nursing is most or least at risk. There is also no information on the choice of specialty as a cause or an effect of impairment.

Environment

Parkes (1982) examined the level of depression and anxiety among British nursing students in medical and surgical rotations and found that higher levels of anxiety and depression were exhibited by students on the medical units. This finding was attributed to differences in the social climate of the two units, as well as to the greater demands of the nurses' involvement with dying and chronically-ill patients in the medical units. This study is very important because it identifies the importance of context in the development of impairment. This type of investigation also raises the issue of occupational stress within nursing. Stress can be an important factor in substance abuse.

Burnout

Normative data on the instruments that measure burnout, a type of occupational stress germane to nursing, are just beginning to appear in the literature, but the prevalence of burnout in practicing nurses is not known nor is the relationship of burnout to impairment.

The data from one investigation on nursing students suggest that there is a relationship between burnout symptoms and increased use of alcohol (Haack, 1987). It is not clear whether the use of alcohol leads to increased burnout or whether alcohol is used to deal with feelings of burnout. Nonetheless, further exploration of the relationship between these variables could lead to the development of primary prevention strategies for students in nursing.

Familial Alcoholism

Several reports indicate that prevalence of children of alcoholics within the helping professions is higher than in the general population (Bissell & Haberman, 1984; Pilat & Jones, 1984). A study of three classes of undergraduates within a college of nursing did not support this assumption. When compared to the general population, there was no difference (Haack & Harford, 1988). On the other hand, studies done on treatment populations do indicate that nurses impaired by alcohol or drugs report more familial alcoholism than does the general population (Norris, 1986; Bissell & Haberman, 1984; Sullivan, 1985). These findings are consistent with other research which provides evidence of a genetic influence in the development of alcoholism. Familial alcoholism is an important risk factor that should be considered in the development of prevention strategies. Other dysfunctions mentioned in the literature that contribute to impairment of practice are depressive disorders, eating disorders, and burnout.

Depression

The prevalence of depressive disorders among nurses is not known. However, since women predominate in the nursing profession and women are more at risk for depression, it is possible that depression is a cause of impairment. One preliminary study on nursing students indicates that depression may indeed be a serious problem within nursing. Fifty-five percent of the students studied scored over the cutoff of 16 on the CES-D depression scale, which indicates risk for clinical depression. Reliable epidemiologic studies estimate that 4 to 10% of the general population suffer from a depressive disorder (NIMH, 1984). When Nigerian and American student nurses were compared, the mean CES-D scores were 16.5 and 18.3 respectively (Haack, 1988; Haack & Harford, 1987). Other studies are needed that investigate the level of depression among students and practicing nurses, using a clinical diagnostic tool that can determine the nature and severity of depression within the profession.

Eating Disorders

Although the existence of eating disorders as a co-morbid state with addictive disorders has been raised in clinical papers, there are no statistics on how widespread this problem is in nursing. The relationship between eating disorders and impairment has not been studied adequately.

Attitudes

Several studies have been done on attitudes of various groups toward aspects of impairment (Hendrix, Sabritt, & McDaniel, 1986; Hughes, 1986a; Long, 1986; Marks, Reed, & Alexander, 1985). In view of nursing history and the influence of Victorian mores, the profession's attitudes toward impaired nurses must be ascertained because they influence the implementation of policies and programs. The best-intentioned policies will be rendered useless in the face of administrators and peers who view impairment as a moral problem instead of a professional issue. In this sense a kind of double standard exists in the profession. While many professionals have little difficulty in seeing their addicted patients as ill people deserving medical care, they may have very punitive attitudes toward their peers with the same problem. A nurse with a drug problem is often perceived by other nurses as different from or less deserving than nurses with other types of medical problems.

Characteristics of Impaired Nurses

The clinical literature contains some descriptions of the characteristics of the impaired nurse. Although these are interesting profiles, clinical impressions must be studied in a systematic way. Sullivan (1987) compared addicted nurses with nonaddicted nurses in regard to gender, familial alcoholism, familial depression, sexual trauma and functioning, sexual preference, parental status, marital history, physical health, depressive illness, and alcoholism in spouse. Men accounted for 12% of the chemically dependent sample but only 2% of the nondependent sample. The chemically dependent nurses reported significantly more family history of alcoholism and depression, more problems in the sexual area (incest, sexual molestation, out-of-wedlock pregnancy, miscarriage, abortion), more homosexual preference, more history of physical illness and depressive illness, more often were parents, and more often married an alcoholic spouse. Although ths study is not representative of the impaired nurse population, it does raise important issues to be studied in future investigations.

Other literature within the social/psychological category on the study of the impaired nurse contains descriptive data on drinking history, use of drugs, suicide attempts, alcohol-related hospitalizations, familial alcoholism, medical history, and self-esteem (Alfano, 1986; Caroselli-Karinja & Zboray, 1986; Doyle, 1985; Halsey, 1985; Royem, 1982). Church (1985) has also provided a historical perspective on the impaired nurse. Although the etiologic complexity of substance-abuse disorders will most likely make it impossible that a profile will fit the characteristics of all impaired nurses, this literature is significant because it identifies risk factors than can guide the development of prevention strategies and provide the database for other studies.

Evaluation Studies

Most of the literature on peer assistance, group treatment, support groups, employee assistance programs, and community-based models describe the components of the various procedures used in assessment, intervention, and referral (Butcher & Talbott, 1984; Curran, 1984; Estes, 1986; Kabb, 1984; O'Conner & Robinson, 1985; Patrick, 1984; Smith & Seymour, 1985). None of the literature describes systematic evaluation of these approaches. For instance, there have been no attempts to systematically compare various intervention approaches or tailor specific treatments to the individual. For example, standardized treatment plans are not adequate for nurses who have a major depressive disorder coexisting with a substance-abuse disorder; they may require a specific type of treatment or series of treatments. Although clinicians may have some idea about what is therapeutically appropriate for such conditions, these interventions need to be tested. Chaisson-Stewart (1988) has begun a preliminary investigation of the efficacy of the Phoenix model which will be a valuable contribution to the field.

The profession is comprised of nurses from different levels of education and training with diverse professional roles. Yet, most studies and articles on impaired practice pertain to the staff nurse. Investigations also need to explore the best approaches to impairment in academe, administration, and public health.

Treatment evaluation studies require a high level of skill in conceptualization, design, and implementation because of the difficulty in controlling for all of the variables. Nonetheless, if the efficacy of prevention and intervention programs is ever to be known, it is imperative that studies attempt to investigate the following questions:

Who is reached by peer assistance networks?
How effective are peer assistance networks?
How effective is the employee assistance programs (EAP) approach?
Who is most effectively reached by EAP programs?
How effective is the community-based model?
How do peer assistance networks, EAPs, and community-based programs compare in terms of the numbers and types of nurses they reach and the outcomes of the interventions they provide?
Is in-patient or out-patient treatment most effective for the impaired nurse?
Or, who is appropriate for in-patient treatment and who is appropriate for out-patient treatment?
Is psychotherapy appropriate for this population?
Is group psychotherapy more effective than individual psychotherapy?
What is the role of self-help groups in recovery?
How effective are self-help groups for this population?
In view of the studies that indicate impaired nurses are more often offspring of an alcoholic parent, do these nurses also need to participate in a self-help group for adult children of alcoholics as well as in Alcoholics Anonymous or Narcotics Anonymous?

Nursing uses the scientific process as a basis for practice. It is essential that the profession not lose sight of this process in its endeavors to help the nurse with impaired functioning caused by substance abuse or psychiatric disorders. Accurate treatment evaluation requires that treatment groups be standardized and randomized, which is difficult without large numbers of subjects and adequate financial resources. Nevertheless, it is possible to collect more reliable and valid data about impairment by using standardized clinical tools such as the Schedule for Affective Disorders and Schizophrenia (SADS) (Endicott & Spitzer, 1978) and published substance-dependence scales (Lettieri, Nelson, & Sayers, 1985). These instruments would be helpful in exploring the complexity of impairment in terms of severity, co-morbidity, and the effectiveness of interventions.

Hendrix and Gray (1987) reported that nurses in their study have been wrongfully accused of substance abuse when the impairment was actually due to other causes. This is an issue that must be addressed in the assessment phase of treatment as well as in the evaluation of the policies developed by most nursing organizations. The resolution which was passed by the House of Delegates at the ANA Convention in 1982 and ultimately became the basis for the ANA policy on impairment called for the establishment of programs of assistance and interventions for nurses whose functioning is impaired due to misuse of alcohol and other drugs or because of emotional and psychological dysfunction.

While the policy of ANA encompasses psychological dysfunction as well as substance dependence, most programs that are operational are designed to meet only the needs of the nurse impaired by the misuse of chemical substances. In order to adequately meet the needs of nurses who are impaired because of psychological dysfunction, the use of tools developed for psychiatric assessment such as the SADS (Endicott & Spitzer, 1978) will be necessary. This, of course, requires an interviewer who is highly skilled and trained. Nevertheless, this type of data from a random sample of impaired nurses who are entering treatment would be invaluable. The benefits of doing so will be two-fold: (1) The interviewer would have a thorough and accurate assessment of the issues involved in impairment, and (2) the use of this sophisticated tool would contribute to a database which will ultimately provide a clearer picture of the impairment in nursing. It may be that the best way to develop an effective evaluation research program on nursing impairment will be for nursing organizations to consolidate efforts in the collection of data that is comparable in terms of the instruments used and the assessment process carried out for each nurse. Programs in Texas and Canada have utilized a battery of standard assessment tools which could serve as models for others (Alexander, 1988, chapter 11 this book).

Policy Studies

The use of drugs and alcohol and the consequences of misuse by nursing students and practicing nurses are influenced to some extent by policies that are created through state legislation, professional organizations, and educational and employing institutions. Studies of policy include policy analysis and policy evaluation (Gerace, 1985; Hughes, 1986b). Mandatory reporting laws and diversion laws and urine and blood screening regulations have been passed by state legislatures, but they vary greatly from state to state. Likewise, most state nursing organizations have some policy or program that addresses impairment issues, but these vary greatly in what services they provide. Ongoing analysis of these policies is essential.

Prevention Studies

There has been a dearth of prevention studies in the substance-abuse field. However, it seems appropriate that investigations of impairment among nursing students is the place to begin. In a longitudinal study on students in nursing school programs conducted by Haack (1988), the data showed that students in the sample were experiencing symptoms of burnout that were comparable to working nurses and that these symptoms increased with years in school. Cross-sectional analyses of the data indicated that emotional exhaustion and depersonalization (cynical attitudes toward patients) were the burnout factors involved. The findings also showed that these students were experiencing a high level of depressive symptomatology, and although numbers of depressive symptoms varied over time, there appeared to be a trend toward a decrease in symptoms as class level increased. This decrease in depressive symptoms paralleled the increase in burnout symptoms, i.e., as students became more unfeeling toward patients, they appeared to become less depressed. Moreover, the findings showed that drinking frequency and total consumption of alcohol increased significantly between sophomore and junior years and remained at that level through the senior year (Haack, 1988). This study also showed a significant relationship between burnout and alcohol consumption (Haack, 1987).

Other analyses of this data revealed that 14% of the nursing students report problems in work or school as a result of alcohol or drug use (Haack & Harford, 1985). This study as well as other literature on nursing students indicate that primary prevention programs are needed in the curriculum of the undergraduate programs (Haack, 1985; Perkins, Daghestani, & Schnoll, 1982; Solari-Twadell, 1982). One such program has been initiated at the University of Tennessee (Greenhill, Skinner, & Smith, 1987). Some extensive work has been done to develop programs of intervention for the individual who is abusing alcohol or drugs but is not alcoholic (Marlatt & Gordon, 1985; Sanchez-Craig, 1984). Interventions based on these models should be adapted to students and practicing nurses and then evaluated.

There is some evidence that supportive interaction with a faculty member does help to decrease the consequences of the stress involved in nursing education. Haack (1988) reported that students who reported positive interactions with peers and faculty were less depressed and less emotionally exhausted (a factor in burnout). In addition, students who reported a sense of internal control over events in their environment had greater feelings of competence. Gardner, Wilshack, and Slotnick (1984) studied medical students and found that a program designed to increase faculty support resulted in reduced student alcohol consumption. These studies suggest that interventions which increase social support between faculty and students might provide some protection against heavier alcohol consumption, some aspects of burnout, and depression. It also suggests that cognitive interventions that teach students how to analyze and gain a sense of control in their environment may be helpful.

Prevention is basic to nursing education and practice, but its importance has not been acknowledged in regard to the issue of impairment. Many of the tertiary intervention programs have been developed after some negative exposure by the media. The need for primary and secondary intervention cannot be dramatized nearly as well. Nevertheless, there is evidence that such initiatives are needed (Brake & Werne, 1982; Cohen & Callahan, 1986; Waits, 1984).

Theoretical Models

Several models have been developed to explain the etiology and development of impairment. A few of these are explored in the literature. Most of what is written is based on an assumption that impairment is a disease, although very little explanation is given as to what that means. Most explanations of the disease model refer to the need for abstinence as a means of gaining control over alcohol or drug use, which pertains more to consequences than to etiology or development. We need to be more precise about how the term disease is defined—especially in light of the recent Supreme Court decision which favors interpretation of the law rather than analyses of scientific data.

Other models that have been used to explain impairment are self-annihilation, Roy's adaptation, stress and attribution (Haack, 1985; Huckabay, 1985; Hutchinson, 1986; Maher, 1986). Hutchinson (1986) conducted interviews and participant observations to generate a substantive-grounded theory that explains the process of nurses becoming chemically dependent. The stages and phases of self-annihilation were defined as initiating, connecting, experimenting, dialogue with self, disengaging, routinizing, craving, and surrendering. These stages are somewhat similar to those described by Jellinek (1952) in his analysis of drinking behavior among male alcoholics. Hutchinson's (1986) analysis provides a qualitative perspective on drug and alcohol dependence among nurses and thus contributes to a deeper understanding of addicted women as well. These models are useful in providing a total explanation for the antecedents, manifestations, and consequences of impairment. Further work must test the application of various models of impaired practice among nurses and nursing students.

Conclusion

There is currently much concern in the United States over the shortage of nurses and the decline in enrollment in nursing schools. It is clear that there are no easy solutions to these problems, which makes the retention of existing nurses more important than ever. The work of Bissell and Haberman (1984) indicates that the impaired professionals in their study were high achieving and valuable members of the professional community before they became ill. If nursing is to advance professionally, it cannot afford to neglect the health and well-being of its members. Although it is clear from this review of the literature that much progress has been made in greater awareness of the problem of impaired practice within nursing, most of this information is documented as papers presented at scientific meetings. It is also clear that the study of impaired practice is still in the early stages. Continued research and more rigorous research is strongly indicated. The need for further work in this area will benefit not only the individual nurse but the patient and the profession as well. Future work should address the following:

1. The scope and severity of impairment within nursing determined by clinical studies using reliable and valid clinical tools.
2. Accurate data on the prevalence of alcohol and drug use among student nurses and practicing nurses.
3. Accurate morbidity data on the prevalence of substance-abuse disorders, eating disorders, depressive disorders, and stress-related disorders such as burnout. These statistics will better define the magnitude of the problem.
4. Accurate data on the cause of death among nurses, especially those deaths related to a substance-abuse disorder or a depressive disorder.
5. Evaluation programs to gain a better understanding of what interventions are most effective for which nurses.
6. Initiation and evaluation of primary, secondary, and tertiary prevention strategies.

In addition, more published studies on nursing impairment issues and the exploration of possibilities for gaining access to large national data sets for secondary analysis, which may contain valuable information on nurses, are needed.

This chapter has attempted to provide an overview of the research on the issue of impairment in nursing. What is known is based largely on clinical wisdom and practical experience. It is understandable why this is so. The nursing profession is based on clinical education and practice. It is the extensive clinical expertise of the members of the profession that guides the present programs of prevention, treatment, and research on the issue of impairment within nursing. Testing the generalizability of these clinical observations and building on the work that has already begun are important tasks before us.

References

Addiction Research Foundation. (1984). *Statistics on Alcohol Use: Data Available by Sept. 1984.* (Nigeria, p. 214, Table 9). Addiction Research Foundation: Toronto.

Alexander, D. (1988, May 12). Texas peer assistance program for impaired nurses. Paper presented at First National Conference on Nursing Impairment and Well-Being. Minneapolis, MN.

Alfano, G. J. (1986, Spring). Why a nurse? *DANA Newsletter,* pp. 2–3.

American Association of Occupational Health Nurses (1986). AAOHN position statement: Impaired nurses. *AAOHN Journal, 34*(4), 183.

American Nurses' Association (May, 1984). *Addictions and psychological dysfunctions in nursing: The profession's response to the problem.* Kansas City, MO.

Billings, C. (1986, March 26–28). *Alcohol consumption practices of North Carolina nurses.* Paper presented at First National Conference for Research and Study on Substance Abuse in Nursing. Atlanta, GA.

Bissell, L., & Haberman, P. W. (1984). *Alcoholism in the professions.* New York: Oxford University Press.

Brake, J. O., & Werne, N. (1982, May). Teaching strategies in substance abuse for student nurses. *Proceedings of Nurse Educator Conference on Alcohol and Drug Abuse* (pp. 138–144). Colorado Springs, CO.

Butcher, T. E., & Talbott, G. D. (1984). Dynamics in group process in impaired health professionals. *Journal of the Medical Association of Georgia. 73*(11), 771–774.

Buxton, M., Jessup, M., & Landry, M. (1985). Treatment of the chemically dependent health professional. In: H. Milkman & H. Shaffer (Eds.), *The Addictions: Multidisciplinary Perspectives and Treatment.* Lexington, MA: Lexington Books.

Caroselli-Karinja, M. F., & Zboray, S. D. (1986). Impaired nurses. *Journal of Psychosocial Nursing and Mental Health Services. 24*(6), 15,16–19.

Chaisson-Stewart, M. (1988, May 13). The phoenix group treatment program: A group psychotherapy model. Paper presented at First National Conference on Nursing Impairment and Well-Being. Minneapolis, MN.

Church, O. M. (1985). Sairey Gamp revisited: A historical inquiry into alcoholism and drug dependency. *Nursing Administration Quarterly, 9*(2), 10–21.

Cohen, S., & Callahan, J. F. (1986). Appendix C: Resources for training the physician and health professional in drugs, alcohol, and prescribing. *Diagnosis and Treatment of Drug and Alcohol Abuse* (pp. 231–292). New York, NY: Haworth Press.

Crowley, T. J. (1984). Contingency contracting treatment of drug-abusing physicians, nurses, and dentists. *NIDA Research Monograph Series 46: Behavioral Intervention Techniques in Drug Abuse Treatment,* 68–83.

Curran, R. F. (1984). Hospital, heal thyself: Coping with impaired providers and other hospital employees. Commentary. *Quality Review Bulletin, 10*(11), 335-339.

Doyle, M. K. (1985, August). Personal and professional self-esteem of addicted nurses. *Proceedings of the 34th International Congress on Alcoholism and Drug Dependence, 2,* 343–346.

Endicott, J., & Spitzer, R. L. (1978). A diagnostic interview: The schedule for affective disorder and schizophrenia. *Archives of General Psychiatry, 35,* 837–844.

Engs, R. C. (1982). Drinking patterns and attitudes toward alcoholism of Australian human-service students. *Journal of Studies on Alcohol, 43*(5), 517–531.

Estes, N. J. (1986). Group treatment of nurses with substance use disorders. In. N. Estes & E. Heinemann (Eds.). *Alcoholism: Development, Consequences and Interventions* (3rd ed.), pp. 283–302. St. Louis: C. V. Mosby.

Florida Nurses Association. (1985). *Nursing administrators guide for the management of substance abuse problems among nurses* [Report, Program Plan (04)]. Orlando, FL.

Gardner, R., Wilsnack, S., & Slotnick, H. (1984). Communication, social support, and alcohol use in first year medical students. *Journal of Studies on Alcohol, 44,* 188–193.

Gerace, L. (1985, August). Analysis of policy and program implementation for the impaired nurse: What is being done in the United States. *Proceedings of the 34th International Congress on Alcoholism and Drug Dependence, 2,* 53–55. Calgary, Canada.

Green, P., (1986). Nursing and its impaired colleagues. *Almacan, 16*(6), 20–21.

Greenhill, E., Skinner, K., & Smith D. (1987, March 25). A peer assistance program for a college of nursing. Paper presented at Fifth National Impaired Nurse Symposium and Research Conference. Atlanta, GA.

Haack, M. R. (1985). *Antecedents of the impaired nurse: Burnout, depression, substance use among student nurses.* Unpublished doctoral dissertation, University of Illinois at Chicago.

Haack, M. R. (1987, April). Alcohol use and burnout among student nurses. *Nursing & Health Care, 8*(4), 239–242.

Haack, M. R. (1988). Stress and impairment among nursing students. *Research in Nursing and Health.*

Haack, M., and Harford, T. (1984). Drinking patterns among student nurses. *The International Journal of the Addictions, 19*(5), 577–583.

Haack, M. R., & Harford, T. C. (1985). Patterns of substance use and response to stress among developing professionals, In H. Parvez, E. Burns, Y. Burov, & S. Parvez (Eds.). *Progress in Alcohol Research,* Vol. 1 (pp. 201–226). Utrecht, Holland: VNU Science Press.

Haack, M., & Harford, T. C. (1987, June 5). A comparative study of drinking and drug use among Nigerian and American student nurses. Paper presented at 33rd International Institute on the Prevention and Treatment of Alcoholism. Lausanne, Switzerland.

Haack, M. R., & Harford, T. C. (1988). Nursing students with alcoholic fathers. *Issues in Mental Health Nursing, 9*(2), 181–188.

Halsey, J. (1985). Moderately troubled nurse: A not-so-uncommon entity. *Nursing Administration Quarterly, 9*(2), 69–76.

Haynes-Streaty, C., & Medina, L. (1985). Impaired nurse treatment: California leads the way. *EAP Digest, 5*(3), 63–65.

Hendrix, M. J., & Gray, N. (1987, March). Nursing impairment and wrongful accusation. Paper presented at Fifth National Impaired Nurse Symposium and Research Conference. Atlanta, GA.

Hendrix, M. J., Sabritt, D., & McDaniel, A. (1986). Nurses assisting nurses: A model for the integration of clinical and professional perspectives in the study of nursing impairment. Presented at *First National Conference for Research and Study on Substance Abuse in Nursing,* Atlanta, GA.

Huckabay, L. M. D. (1985). Troubled nurse: A conceptual framework for resolving problems. *Nursing Administration Quarterly, 9*(2), 22–30.

Hughes, T. (1986a). Chemical impairment in nursing: Attitudes and perceptions of first-level nursing administrators. Unpublished manuscript.

Hughes, T. (1986b, June). Chemical impairment in nursing: Policy and program implementation. Paper presented at 32nd International Institute on the Prevention and Treatment of Alcoholism. Budapest, Hungary.

Hutchinson, S. (1986, July/August). Chemically dependent nurses: The trajectory toward self-annihilation. *Nursing Research, 35*(4), 196–201.

Jellinek, E. M. (1952). Phases of alcohol addiction. *Quarterly Journal of Studies in Alcohol,* 13:673–684.

Kaab, G. M. (1984). Chemical dependency; Helping your staff. *Journal of Nursing Administration, 14*(11), 18–23.

Katz, R. M. (1983). Causes of death among registered nurses. *Journal of Occupational Medicine, 25*(10), 760–762.

Kizer, K. W., Kelter, A., Lera, G., Mitchell, D. W., & Doebbert, G. (1987, March). Female mortality by occupation. *California Occupational Mortality 1979-1981,* 83–84,170–171.

Lettieri, D., Nelson, J., & Syers, M. (1985). *Treatment Handbook Series 2: Alcoholism Treatment Assessment Research Instruments,* National Institute of Alcohol Abuse and Alcoholism [DHHA Publication No. (ADM) 85-1380.] Washington, D.C.: U.S. Government Printing Office.

Long, P. (1986). Effect of an alcoholism education program on student nurses' attitudes toward alcoholism. *Dissertation Abstracts International, 46*(12), 3610A.

Maher, L. J. (1986). *Recovering impaired nurses: A follow-up study.* Unpublished doctoral dissertation, Emory University, School of Nursing, Atlanta.

Marks, L. N., Reed, J. C., & Alexander, D. (1985). Attitudes of nurses affecting the rehabilitation of impaired nurses using and abstaining from drugs and alcohol. *Proceedings of the 34th International Congress on Alcoholism and Drug Dependence,* Calgary, Alberta, Canada, 2, 67–68.

Marlatt, G. A., & Gordon, J. R. (1985). *Relapse Prevention: Maintenance Strategies in the Treatment of Addictive Behaviors.* New York: Guilford Press.

McAuliffe, W. E., Wechsler, H., Rohman, M., Soboroff, S. H., Fishman, P., Toth, D., and Friedman, R. (1984, March). Psychoactive drug use by young and future physicians. *Journal of Health and Social Behavior, 25*(1), 34–54.

Milham, S., Jr. (1983). Occupational mortality in Washington State 1950–1979 (NIOSH Research Report) (HEW Publication No. 76-175-A-C). Washington, D.C.: U.S. Department of Health and Human Services.

NIMH, U.S. Department of Health and Human Services. (1984). *Depression: What we know.* [DHHS Publication No. (ADM) 85-1318]. Washington, D.C.: Author.

Norris, J. (1986). Critical factors associated with substance abuse and chemical dependency in nurse anesthesia. *Presentation at the 1st National Conference for Research and Study on Substance Abuse in Nursing.* Atlanta, GA.

O'Connor, P., & Robinson, R. S. (1985). Managing impaired nurses. *Nursing Administration Quarterly, 9*(2), 1–9.

O'Connor, P., Robinson, R. S., Ferrara, E. R., et. al. (1985). On the scene: The troubled nurse at the University of Cincinnati Hospital. *Nursing Administration Quarterly, 9*(2), 31–68.

Parkes, K. R. (1982). Occupational stress among student nurses: A natural experiment. *Journal of Applied Psychology, 67*(6), 784–796.

Patrick, P. K. S. (1984). Self-preservation: Confronting the issue of nurse impairment. *Journal of Substance Abuse Treatment, 1*(2), 99–105.

Perkins, E. J., Daghestani, A. N., & Schnoll, S. H. (1982, May). Substance abuse among nurses: Curriculum as a primary preventive strategy. *Proceedings of Nurse Educator Conference on Alcohol and Drug Abuse* (pp. 106–121). Colorado Springs, CO.

Pilat, J. M., & Jones, J. W. (Winter, 1984–85). Identification of children of alcoholism: Two empirical studies. *Alcohol Health & Research World, 9*(2), 27–36.

The Registrar General's Decennial Supplement for England and Wales, 1970–1972. *Occupational Mortality,* Series DS No. 1. London.

Riche, W., Rudnick, P., Epstein, J. (Producers), & Anstaugh, D. (Director). (1986). *Deadly Care* (Made for T.V. Movie). Universal Television Los Angeles.

Royem, D. D. (1982). Nurse who abuses alcohol. *Proceedings of Nurse Educator Conference on Alcohol and Drug Abuse, pp.* 122–128.

Sanchez-Craig, M. (1984). *A Therapist's Manual for Secondary Prevention of Alcohol Problems.* Toronto: Addiction Research Foundation.

Smith, D. C., & Seymour, R. (1985). Clinical approach to the impaired health professional. *The International Journal of the Addictions, 20*(5), 713–722.

Solari-Twadell, P. A. (1982, May). Student nurses with alcohol and/or drug problems: The response of the educator. *Proceedings of Nurse Educator Conference on Alcohol and Drug Abuse* (pp. 129–136). Colorado Springs, CO.

State of California, Department of Health Services, Health Demographics Section, Occupational Mortality Study File. 1980 census sample.

Sullivan, E. J. (1985, August). Alcohol and drug impairment in registered nurses. *Proceedings of the 34th International Congress on Alcoholism and Drug Dependence, 2,* 16–18. Calgary, Canada.

Sullivan, E. J. (1987). Comparison of chemically dependent and nonchemically-dependent nurses on familial, personal and professional characteristics. *Journal of Studies on Alcohol, 48,* 563–568.

Waits, R. J. (1984). Hospital-based wellness committee. *Journal of the Medical Association of Georgia, 73*(11), 779–780.

Appendix I: Impaired Nurse Program Activities of State Nurses' Associations*

During May 1984, and again in December 1984, January 1986, March 1987 and April 1988, the state nurses' associations, constituents of the American Nurses' Association, had an opportunity to describe program activities in their states related to the problem of nurses whose practice is impaired by addiction or psychological dysfunction. Following are program descriptions submitted by state nurses' associations.

Alabama State Nurses' Association

An Ad Hoc Committee on Peer Assistance was appointed by the ASNA Board of Directors to investigate and recommend a course of action regarding peer assistance. This committee was formed as the result of a resolution regarding chemical dependency among nurses, which was adopted by the ASNA House of Delegates in 1983. The Ad Hoc Committee has referred this issue to the Psychiatric and Mental Health Nursing Council.

Alaska Nurses Association

The Alaska Nurses Association has developed guidelines for a peer assistance program entitled "New Directions." Currently, educational activities are under way. For the actual implementation of its program, AaNA is looking into combining efforts with other health care providers (physicians, pharmacists, dentists) to help overcome the difficulties of reaching impaired professionals

*Compiled by the American Nurses' Association, 1988.

in outlying bush communities. The Alaska Board of Nursing has adopted its own position statement regarding the needs of substance abusive nurses, and is supportive of AaNA's efforts. In addition, a local chapter of Nurses House has been established in Anchorage.

Contact: Gail McGuill, R.N.
Alaska Nurses Association
237 East Third Avenue
Anchorage, AK 99501
(907) 274-0827 (daytime)

Arizona Nurses' Association

The Arizona Nurses' Association Impaired Nurse Committee is involved in the following activities to assist impaired nurses: (1) conducts needs assessment; (2) works with the Arizona State Board of Nursing and agencies with assistance programs and with nurses who work in chemical dependency to develop criteria for identifying the impaired nurse; (3) developed a model for confrontation and intervention; (4) maintains an ongoing list of treatment facilities; (5) presents workshops to educate other nurses; and (6) compiles educational information on ethical/legal issues.

Contact: Sarah Withcott, M.S., R.N.
Chairperson, Impaired Nurse Committee
Arizona Nurses' Association
1850 East Southern Avenue, Suite 1
Tempe, AZ 85282
(602) 831-0404 (daytime)

Arkansas State Nurses' Association

District 10, ASNA has established the Nurses for Recovery Task Force. The following are objectives that have been met or are in progress: A support group for recovering nurses meets weekly; philosophy, policies, and job descriptions are written; collaboration ongoing with the state board of nursing; grant writing and development of educational programs are in progress.

Contact: Charlene Bradham, M.N.Sc, R.N.
Department of Nursing
University of Arkansas-Little Rock
2801 S. University Avenue
Little Rock, AS 72204

(501) 569-8084 or 661-6090
7:00 a.m.-3:00 p.m., Mon.-Fri.
(501) 562-2444 or 663-2363
4:00 p.m.-6:00 a.m.

California Nurses Association

The California Nurses Association established a Well Being Committee to assist nurses with chemical dependency and stress as it relates to their work. The committee members are knowledgeable in the area of drug and alcohol addiction, mental health and legal issues. The purpose is to educate nurses, nursing service directors and hospital administration regarding these problems.

Contact: Connie Davis, R.N.
Chairperson, Well Being Committee
California Nurses Association
1855 Folsom Street, Suite 670
San Francisco, CA 94103
(415) 864-4141 (daytime)

Colorado Nurses Association

Colorado Nurses Association houses N.U.R.S.E.S. of Colorado Corporation which is a separate corporate entity. N.U.R.S.E.S. (Nurses United for Recovery, Support, and Education Successfully) of Colorado Corporation is a peer employee assistance program providing assessment, referral, peer intervention, monitoring/follow-up, support groups, training/consultation, and confidential information phone line 24 hours/day.

Contact: Elizabeth M. Pace, B.S., R.N.
Executive Director
N.U.R.S.E.S. of Colorado Corporation
P.O. Box 61294
Denver, CO 80206
(303) 758-0596
8:00 a.m.-4:00 p.m.; Mon.-Fri.
Hotline: (303) 758-0596. This is an answering service, available 24 hours every day.

Connecticut Nurses' Association

The Connecticut Nurses' Association's Peer Assistance Network for Nurses currently has educational and (limited) referral programs. These programs are presently being re-evaluated by the CNA Board of Directors and the Network.

Contact: Beatrice R. Burns, M.S.N., R.N., C.S.
Chairperson, Peer Assistance Network for Nurses
C/O Connecticut Nurses Association
1 Prestige Drive
Meriden, CT 06450
(203) 238-1207 (daytime)

Delaware Nurses' Association

The Impaired Nurse Hotline has been in existence since December, 1986. Volunteers are prepared to conduct crisis intervention, refer nurses whose lives are affected by substance abuse or mental health problems to treatment/rehabilitation programs, and to offer appropriate support.

Contact: L. Alberta Regan, M.S.N., R.N.
Chairperson, Impaired Nurse Peer Assistance Committee
2109 Milltown Road
Wilmington, DE 19808
(302) 454-3942 (daytime)
(302) 994-5638 (evening)
Hotline: (302) 366-1775. This is an answering service, available 24 hours every day.

District Of Columbia Nurses' Association, Inc.

The District of Columbia Nurses' Association offers educational programs, makes available resource materials and refers nurses with addiction problems to treatment programs. Peer review legislation that will make possible intervention through the professional association will be introduced in 1988. DCNA's intervention activities will begin following successful passage of that legislation.

Contact: Evelyn Sommers, M.B.A.
Executive Director, District of Columbia Nurses' Association, Inc.
Suite 306
5100 Wisconsin Avenue, N.W.
Washington, D.C. 20016
(212) 244-2705

Florida Nurses Association

The Florida Nurses Association Council on Chemical Dependency provides nurses interested in, or working in the field of addiction, with a statewide organization to address current issues, continuing education and networking. The activity of Council members is focused on educating nurses and nursing students about the Board of Nursing's Intervention Project for Nurses (in lieu of disciplinary proceedings) and treatment resources as well as identification and education of the "at risk" nurse or student and appropriate management, including standardized curriculum in nursing programs.

Contact: Joyce Dorner, R.N.
Chairperson, Council on Chemical Dependency
Florida Nurses Association
P.O. Box 536985
Orlando, FL 32853-6985
(407) 896-3261 (daytime)

Georgia Nurses Association, Inc.

The overall goal of the Georgia Nurses Association Impaired Nurse Committee is to identify and assist impaired nurses to seek treatment for addictive diseases so they can remain useful members of our profession. We provide information, referral, intervention, support groups, education, consultation and advocacy when the need is identified.

Contact: Rose Johnson, M.S.N., R.N.
Chairperson, Impaired Nurse Committee
277 Ashtonwood Drive
Marinez, GA 30907,
or
Georgia Nurses Association
1362 West Peachtree, N.W.
Atlanta, GA 30309
(404) 828-2079 (Ms. Johnson-daytime)
(404) 863-7383 (evening)
(404) 876-4624 (GNA)
Hotline: (404) 876-8416. This is an answer phone, available 24 hours every day. Rose Johnson responds to these call personally, or refers them to district advocates.

Hawaii Nurses' Association

A peer assistance committee is established to provide information/education/ referral to nurses or their employers.

Contact: Sunny Thompson, R.N.
Committee Chairperson
1720 Ala Moana Blvd., Suite 807B
Honolulu, HI 96815
(808) 947-1635 (daytime/evng.)

Idaho Nurses Association

The Idaho Nurse Peer Assistance Program provides education, awareness and practices which promote prevention, early intervention and support strategies for nurses and their patients at high risk for chemical dependency.

Contact: Joan Nelson, R.N.
1010 North Orchard
Boise, ID 83706, or
Idaho Nurses Association
200 North 4th Street, Suite 20
Boise, ID 83702-6001
(208) 377-8204 (Ms. Nelson-daytime)
(208) 345-0500 (INA-daytime)
Hotline: (208) 345-0500. Available 8:00 a.m.-5:00 p.m., Monday-Friday

Illinois Nurses Association

The Illinois Nurses' Association developed a support network for nurses whose professional performance is hampered by abuse of chemicals or any mental or resulting physical illness. This support network is the Peer Assistance Network for Nurses (P.A.N.N.). P.A.N.N. was incorporated as a foundation on November 13, 1987.

Contact: Monica M. Russell, B.S.N., Ed., R.N.
Associate Administrator
Illinois Nurses' Association
20 North Wacker Drive, Suite 2520
Chicago, IL 60606
(312) 236-9708 (daytime)

Indiana State Nurses' Association

The Peer Review and Assistance Program for Registered Nurses is a network of support, monitoring and referral for treatment to nurses whose professional performance is hampered by alcohol and/or other drug abuse, mental dysfunction or physical dysfunction.

Contact: Ernest C. Klein, Jr.
Assistant Director,
Indiana State Nurses' Association
2915 North High School Road
Indianapolis, IN 46224
(317) 299-4575 (daytime)
Hotline: (317) 299-4575. 24 hours every day, on answering machine.

Iowa Nurses' Association

Iowa Nurses' Association has established a Peer Assistance Program Planning Committee. A three-component design is in process: prevention, education, and intervention. Whether the program will be implemented depends on funding.

Contact: Marcene Moran, R.N.
Chairperson, Peer Assistance Program Planning Committee
2525 Apache Drive
Sioux City, IA 51104
(712) 279-2446 (daytime)

Kansas State Nurses Association

Kansan State Nurses Association's Peer Assistance Program works to find and refer nurses (RN's and LPN's) impaired by use of drugs and/or alcohol into treatment and provides intervention, monitoring, education, urine testing and collegial support through the recovery process.

Contact: LaWanda Aarnes, R.N.
Program Director
Peer Assistance Program,
or
Terri Roberts, J.D., R.N.
Executive Director
Kansas State Nurses Association
820 Quincy
Topeka, KS 66612
(913) 233-8638 (KSNA-daytime)

Hotline: none established, but members of committee can be called at anytime:

Pat Green, M.S.W., R.N.
Lawrence, KS
Work (816) 254-3652
Home (913) 842-3893

Sr. Mary Theresa Morris, R.N.
801 South 8th
Atchison, KS 66002

John Aker, M.S., C.R.N.A.
3417 S.W. Birchwood
Topeka, KS 66614
Work (913) 588-6612

Kentucky Nurses Association

Nurses Assisting Nurses (NAN) is sponsored by the University of Kentucky College of Nursing in cooperation with the Kentucky Nurses Association and the Kentucky Board of Nursing. The project consists of clinical counseling services, advocacy, public and professional education, and a longitudinal research study. Services are provided by doctoral and masters-prepared psychiatric/mental health nurses.

Contact: Melva Jo Hendrix, D.N.Sc., R.N.
Professor and Project Director, NAN
University of Kentucky
College of Nursing
800 Rose Street
Lexington, KY 40536
(606) 257-1587 (daytime/evening)
Hotline: (606) 257-1587. Answering service available 24 hours every day.

Louisiana State Nurses Association

The Louisiana State Nurses Association statewide program (LaNNIP-Louisiana Nurses' Network for the Impaired Professional) provides for (1) early detection and identification of impaired nurses or potentially impaired nurses; (2) confrontation of and intervention with such nurses; (3) the evaluation of the conditions underlying their impairment; and (4) assistance in identifying, securing and pursuing effective treatment. Nurses are monitored for two years in practice and in their recovery program.

Contact: Bobby G. Huskey, M.A., B.S.N., R.N.
Chairperson, LSNA Impaired Nurse Committee
Louisiana State Nurses Association
712 Transcontinental Drive
Metairie, LA 70001
(504) 889-1030 (daytime); 568-4203 (daytime); 738-0281 (evening)

Maine State Nurses' Association

The Maine State Nurses' Association has been involved with (1) testifying before the Maine legislature on bills relating to substance abuse (i.e., random drug testing and establishment of employee assistance programs); (2) negotiating contract language for the establishment of employee assistance programs; (3) pursuing a grant to study the needs ot Maine nurses regarding the extensiveness of the problem; (4) license protection; (5) client protection; and (6) the establishment of an impaired nurse program which will educate the public, nurses, related health professionals and employees. The program will include treatment, referral, monitoring, and support and appropriate legislation.

Contact: Anna Gilmore, R.N.
Executive Director
Maine State Nurses' Association
P.O. Box 2240
Augusta, ME 04330
(207) 622-1057 (daytime)

Maryland Nurses Association, Inc.

The Maryland Nurses Association Impaired Nurses Committee recognizes that impaired nursing practice impacts on the individual, the patient, and the nursing profession. It is committed to addressing the problem through education, information sharing, and networking with other groups and professions. It supports referral of a nurse into treatment and rehabilitation. The Committee has supported and encouraged the development of a peer support group, "Nurses Recovering Together"; has developed a state-wide directory of information and referral resources; provides committee sponsored speakers to assist with in-service presentations, staff development and conference planning; participates in interdisciplinary networks through the Professional Rehabilitation Council and national networks; has a pamphlet which is designed to provide information for referral, identification, and education as well as describe the committee's services and activities; and has active involvement with the Maryland Board of Nursing.

Contact: Marie C. McCarthy, M.S., R.N., C.S.
Chairperson, MNA Impaired Nurses Committee
401 Kensington Road
Baltimore, MD 21229
(301) 233-3342 (daytime/evng.) (answering machine)
Hotline: No 24-hour hotline has been established. Call (301) 242-7300 for information and referral resources.

Massachusetts Nurses Association

The Massachusetts Nurses Association Peer Assistance Program is designed to provide support, intervention, and referral through a network of peer assistants—nurse volunteers who know about the disease of chemical dependency and can offer care and concern to the nurse experiencing drug/alcohol problems. The program provides information and support to the nurse manager who has questions regarding chemical dependency.

Contact: Department of Nursing Staff
Massachusetts Nurses Association
340 Turnpike Street
Canton, MA 02021
(617) 821-4625 (daytime)

Michigan Nurses Association

MNA did not establish a peer assistance program of its own, as NPAN (Nurses Peer Assistance Network, Inc.) was established as a non-profit corporation and MNA chose to become a charter member with the goal to support and monitor the effectiveness of the program. However, by mid-1988, NPAN had ceased providing peer assistance support to nurses and MNA is currently actively exploring mechanisms to assure that nurses in Michigan will have access to peer assistance support.

The Michigan Nurses Association's Impaired Professional Functioning Committee has adopted the following goals: 1) Educate the profession on the extent and nature of chemical dependency, 2) Disseminate research on the problem, 3) Ensure the availability of peer assistance programs, and 4) Introduce legislation which would facilitate voluntary suspension of licenses for nurses entering treatment programs. The March, 1987 issue of the *Michigan Nurse* was devoted entirely to the problem of chemical dependency in nursing. It continues to be used as a resource for concerned nurses in the state.

The Michigan Department of Licensing and Regulation has distributed a study of drug diversion by nurses in hospitals. This study documents the extensiveness of the problem of chemical dependency, and is expected to lend support to MNA's proposed licensure legislation.

Contact: Carol E. Franck, M.S.N., R.N.
Executive Director, Michigan Nurses Association
120 Spartan Avenue
East Lansing, MI 48823
(517) 337-1653 (daytime)

Minnesota Nurses Association

The Minnesota Nurses Association's Peer Assistance Program for Nurses has the following components: (1) *referral:* nurses with chemical abuse/dependency problems are followed by the Regional Liaison Person (RLP) from the intervention through 1-2 years into recovery; (2) *education:* speakers are provided at every opportunity to educate others about the problem of chemical dependency; (3) *consultation:* assistance is provided to anyone with questions or concerns about chemical dependency; (4) *back to work issues:* work with receiving staffs and assistance with the development of return to work contracts is provided.

Contact: Lou Erickson, M.P.H., R.N.
Staff Specialist, Nursing Practice
Minnesota Nurses Association
1295 Bandana Boulevard North

St. Paul, MN 55108
(612) 646-4807 (daytime)

Mississippi Nurses' Association

The Mississippi Nurses' Foundation's Educational Resource Committee is offering educational and referral services throughout the state. Nurses seeking assistance are encouraged to call for more information at (601) 982-9183. As a healing and preventative profession, nursing has a commitment to educate the public, peers, and colleagues of the disease concept, rehabilitation, and reentry of those who are chemically dependent.

Contact: David Allday, R.N., C., C.C.R.N.
Chairperson, Educational Resource Committee
Mississippi Nurses' Foundation
135 Bounds Street
Jackson, MS 39206
(601) 982-9183 (daytime)

Missouri Nurses Association

The Missouri Nurses Association Peer Assistance Program was formally incorporated into the association bylaws in 1983. The MONA is now refocusing its Peer Assistance Program. Committee members have been appointed to develop a method to provide support to nurses who are chemically impaired or nurses who are in need of assistance in this area. Other activities will be to develop educational programs for nurses and others on chemical impairment and to provide a telephone number for informational purposes on chemical impairment and/or treatment centers in the state.

Contact: Ann Kellett, J.D., R.N.
Executive Director, Missouri Nurses Association
P.O. Box 325
206 East Dunklin Street
Jefferson City, MO 65102
(314) 636-9576 (daytime)

Montana Nurses' Association

The Montana Nurses' Association affiliated Program for Recovering Nurses (PRN) serves four purposes: 1) To assist nurses (RNs and LPNs) who have been identified as needing rehabilitation into treatment programs, 2) To educate health care workers and the public about the Montana Program for Recovering Nurses, 3) To provide aftercare through a recovery contract for monitoring recovery, and 4) To provide a support group for nurses in recovery.

A task force has been developed to support the introduction of bills into the upcoming legislative session to allocate funds for a diversion program for nurses and to establish limited licensure guidelines for nurses in recovery.

Contact: Carol Sem, B.S.N., R.N.
Program Director
127 North Higgins
Suite H
Missoula, MT 59802
(406) 721-4610 This is an answer phone, available 24 hours every day.

Nebraska Nurses' Association

Nebraska Nurses' Association has an Impaired Nurse Committee and support group in place. The committee has held educational sessions for nurses and has planned a workshop for directors of nursing for the end of April, 1988. Volunteers work with nurses reported to the group, and also work with nurses' employers and monitoring during recovery.

Contact: Kathy Wright, R.N.
Chairperson, NNA Impaired Nurse Program
University of Nebraska Medical Center
NICU
42nd and Dewey
Omaha, Nebraska 68105
(402) 559-5815
7:00 a.m.-4:00 p.m.
(402) 551-4023
4:00 p.m.-7:00 p.m.

Nevada Nurses' Association

The Peer Assistance Committee is composed of volunteer members who hold support group meetings, and are available for one-on-one private counseling. Educational seminars may also be held, for impaired and unimpaired nurses.

Contact: Ardis Kinney, R.N.
Peer Assistance Committee
1315 Westwood Avenue
Reno, NV 89509
(702) 785-6102
8:00 a.m.-4:00 p.m.
(702) 786-5988 (evening) Mon.-Fri. or call NNA office: (702) 825-3555

Group facilitators for support groups—*Nurses Helping Nurses:*
Reno—Mary: (702) 323-0250
Las Vegas—Rosemary: (702) 369-2883

Hotline: (702) 825-3555 Available 9:00 a.m.-3:00 p.m., Monday-Friday.

New Hampshire Nurses' Association

The Nurses' Peer Assistance Group began its work in 1985. It has provided education and information to a variety of nursing groups. On an individual basis, Peer Assistance Group members provide consultation and referral for impaired nurses. Volunteers with the group include both recovering nurses and substance abuse treatment nurses. The volunteer group is very small and informal in nature, and hopes to increase in membership, in order to be able to better serve the needs of New Hampshire nurses. Recovering nurses, substance abuse treatment nurses, and interested others in the profession are all encouraged to become involved.

Contact: Lonnie Larrow, M.S., R.N.
Nurses' Peer Assistance Group
New Hampshire Nurses' Association
48 West Street
Concord, NH 03301
(603) 225-3783

New Jersey State Nurses Association

All impairment calls are handled confidentially and quickly. The nature of the call determines the resources utilized. Education continues to be a major focus of the committee. A *Resource Directory* for New Jersey nurses has been published. The committee continues to seek funding for impairment activities. Peer support groups have been developed.

Contact: Dorothy Flemming
Deputy Director, New Jersey State Nurses Association
320 West State Street
Trenton, NJ 08618
(609) 392-4884 (daytime/evng.)

Hotline: (609) 392-4884. Available 24 hours every day; on tape evenings and weekends.

New Mexico Nurses Association

CAN Recover—Committee to Assist Nurses Recover—provides intervention and referral for nurses with chemical addiction. Confidential and anonymous. Also, conducting educational seminars about chemical dependency among nurses.

Contact: Judith Brown, M.S.N., R.N.
Executive Director, New Mexico Nurses Association
525 San Pedro N.E., Suite 100
Albuquerque, NM 87108
(505) 268-7744 (daytime)
Hotline: (505) 293-5146, available 9:00 a.m.-5:00 p.m., Monday-Friday.
We do not provide crisis service.

New York State Nurses Association

The Committee on Impaired Nursing Practice focuses on education and encouraging peer assistance activities. DNA 1 (Buffalo) has "Nurses Helping Nurses"; DNA 9 (Albany) has "Support Group for Chemically Dependent Nurses"; DNA 14 (Long Island) has "The Committee for the Prevention of Chemically Impaired Nursing Practice." Materials are available on peer assistance, the state of New York's Impaired Professionals Program, hospital-based employee assistance programs and an extensive literature review.

Contact: Gail K. DeMarco, M.S., R.N.
Associate Director, Nursing Practice and Services
New York State Nurses Association
2113 Western Avenue
Guilderland, NY 12084
(518) 456-5371 (daytime)

North Carolina Nurses Association

The North Carolina Nurses Association Peer Assistance Program (PAP) focuses on education regarding the hazards of substance abuse and services to impaired nurses. Four continuing education programs have been developed, and a resource referral file listing services available at facilities in the state has been compiled. Guidelines and an orientation for volunteers have been developed and implemented.

Contact: Janice Millns, M.S.N., R.N.
Assistance Director, North Carolina Nurses Association
P.O. Box 12025
Raleigh, NC 27605
(919) 821-4250
9:30 a.m.-1:30 p.m.; Mon.-Fri.

North Dakota Nurses' Association

The North Dakota Nurses' Association Task Force on the Impaired Nurse has prepared a handbook entitled *Chemical Dependency and the Professional Nurse: A Resource Guide,* which was distributed to all health care facilities in the state. Copies are available at the NDNA office for a fee of $5.00. North Dakota Nurses' Association is currently working with eight other health related professions in the North Dakota Coalition for the Impaired Professional. This organization aspires to facilitate intervention and follow-up for the impaired health professional. Recent legislation has mandated that a $1.00 surcharge be assessed on every nursing licensure fee, and this money will be used to support the coalition's impaired professionals program.

Contacts: Christeen M. Curran, M.S., R.N., C., L.A.C.
Chairperson, Task Force on the Impaired Nurse
or
Nola Helm, R.N.
North Dakota Nurses' Association
Ms. Curran:
1012 16th Street, North
Fargo, ND 58102
(701) 232-5579 (Ms. Curran) (daytime)
or
North Dakota Nurses' Association
212 North Fourth Street
Bismarck, ND 58501
(702) 223-1385 (NDNA) (1:00-5:00 p.m.)

Ohio Nurses Association

The Ohio Nurses Association's Peer Assistance Program for Nurses is a volunteer program that provides intervention, referral and support services to registered nurses who are chemically dependent or physically or mentally impaired. Nurses in the program are monitored for at least two years. Volunteers also assist nurses re-entering the job market.

Contact: Carol A. Jenkins, M.S., R.N.
Director, Nursing Practice
Ohio Nurses Association
4000 East Main Street
Columbus, OH 43213-2950
(614) 237-5414 (daytime), or 475-9745 (evening)

Oklahoma Nurses Association

The Oklahoma Nurse Assistance Program, Inc., was established to provide assistance for licensed nurses at risk for chemical dependence. The program is focused on prevention (continuing education) and intervention and referral.

Contact: Frances I. Waddle, M.S.N., R.N.
Executive Director, Oklahoma Nurses Association

6414 North Santa Fe, Suite A
Oklahoma City, OK 73116
(405) 840-3478 (daytime)
Hotline: (405) 556-4152. Available 24 hours per day.

Oregon Nurses Association

The Oregon Nurses Association founded the Nurse Assistance Network (NAN) as a peer referral and advocacy service offered to: 1. Oregon nurses (R.N., L.P.N., S.N.) experiencing problems with chemical addiction or emotional distress; 2. Employers and colleagues concerned about the problems of nurses in the work setting; 3. Family members who want to help a troubled nurse.

Contact: Ginny Pecora, R.N.
Chairperson, Nurse Assistance Network Committee
616 East 16th
Eugene, OR 97401 (work)
2825 Greentree Way
Eugene, OR 97405 (home)
(503) 687-1110 (daytime); 687-9429 (evening)
Hotline: (503) 243-1244 (Portland); 683-0120 (Eugene). Answering Service available 24 hours per day.

Pennsylvania Nurses Association

The Impaired Nurse Program has engaged in a series of educational programs, audio-visuals, brochures, and a manual to raise awareness of the problem. We are supporting development of recovering nurse support groups, information bureaus, assistance with interventions, referrals, and re-entry. We have worked legislatively to promote a more effective approach to impaired nurses by the state board.

Contact: Jessie F. Igou, Dr.P.H., R.N.
Nursing Practice Director,
PA Nurses Association
2578 Interstate Drive
P.O. Box 8525
Harrisburg, PA 17105-8525
(717) 657-1222 (daytime)

Rhode Island State Nurses' Association

The Rhode Island State Nurses' Association Peer Assistance Program is being professionally managed and staffed by the Rhode Island Employee Assistance Program. Services offered: assessment, referral to treatment, advocacy, aftercare planning, referral to peer support and self-help groups, and monitoring of reentry. Conducts educational programs. Problem areas: alcoholism, drug addiction, emotional problems, marital and family problems, single parenting issues.

Contact: Lorraine Hall, R.N., C.S.
c/o Rhode Island Employee Assistance Program
33 College Hill Road
Warwick, RI 02886
(401) 828-9560 (daytime/evng.)
(answering machine)
Hotline: (401) 828-9560. This is an answer phone only, available 24 hours/day.

South Carolinas Nurses' Association

The Peer Assistance Program for Chemically Dependent Nurses (PAPIN) is a volunteer advocacy program designed to assist nurses with alcohol and/or other drug problems. Major components of the program are education, intervention to facilitate entry into treatment, and peer support throughout treatment and recovery with advocacy for reentry into nursing practice. Peer support groups have been established in regions throughout the state.

Contact: (Ms.) Lloyd Lachicotte, M.S.N., R.N.
Chairperson, Peer Assistance Program for Chemically Dependent Nurses
South Carolina Nurses' Association
1821 Gadsden Street
Columbia, SC 29201
(803) 252-4781 (SCNA-daytime); 734-7758 (Ms. Lachicotte-daytime)

South Dakota Nurses' Association

The South Dakota Nurses' Association supports the efforts of the South Dakota Board of Nursing on behalf of nurses whose practice is impaired by substance abuse.

Tennessee Nurses' Association

The Tennessee Nurses' Association Peer Assistance Program for Chemically Dependent Nurses is an advocacy program to assist nurses in recognizing and seeking treatment for chemical dependency. Strict confidentiality is maintained. After completion of treatment, a two-year follow-up program is required of the recovering nurse.

Contact: Louise Browning, C.A.E.
Executive Director, Tennessee Nurses' Association
1720 West End Building, Suite 400
Nashville, TN 37203
(615) 321-0455 (daytime/evng.)
Hotline: (615) 321-0455. 24 hours every day. On tape evenings and weekends.

Texas Nurses Association

Texas Peer Assistance Program for Impaired Nurses (TPAPIN) is an advocacy program implemented to assist licensed nurses whose practice is impaired by drug or alcohol abuse or by mental illness by allowing the opportunity for rehabilitation before their license is revoked. Confidentiality is strictly maintained. A two-year follow-up program is required of each recovering nurse.

Contact: Andrea Brooks, R.N.
Program Director, Texas Nurses Association
300 Highland Mall Boulevard, Suite 300
Austin, TX 78752-3718
(512) 467-7027 (daytime)
Hotline: (800) 288-5528 (inside Texas only) Available 24 hours/day.

Utah Nurses' Association

The Utah Nurses' Association sponsors Nurses Assisting Nurses with Substance Abuse (NANSA). The program assists nurses identified by the State Board of Nursing or referred directly to UNA with legal, professional, and treatment issues.

Contact: Nadine Ward, M.Sc., R.N.
NANSA Coordinator, Utah Nurses' Association
1058A East 900 South
Salt Lake City, UT 84105
(801) 322-3439 (daytime)

Vermont State Nurses' Association

The charge to the Task Force on Impairment Among Nurses was re-defined by the Vermont State Nurses Association at its Fall, 1986, annual meeting, with the adoption of a resolution. This resolution directed the task force to develop an educational program addressing impairment among nurses and to move forward in the development of a peer support program. The task force has assisted with the development of management principles for dealing with substance abusing health care professionals, and is currently developing a three-hour educational program to be shared with nurses around the state when completed. The task force has received a small community grant from the state Office of Alcohol and Drug Abuse, and is currently working with other state groups to develop a state-wide impairment support program to assist physicians, dentists, veterinarians, pharmacists and nurses whose practice is impaired by substance abuse.

Contact: Executive Director
Vermont State Nurses' Association
500 Dorset Street
South Burlington, VT 05403
(802) 864-9390 (daytime)

Virginia Nurses' Association

The Virginia Nurses' Association's Peer Assistance for Chemically Dependent Nurses Committee provides peer support/advocacy, education, consultation and referral services. Information for wide distribution as handouts have been developed which include a Fact Sheet, Selection Criteria for Treatment Programs, Bibliography and Re-entry Guidelines. This year multiple training programs have been conducted for the Peer Assistance Volunteers who will form the cadre of peer intervenors and monitors of proposed Regional Liaison Teams. The Peer Assistance Volunteer Program has been very well received around the state.

Contact: Lee Crigler, M.S.N., R.N., C.S.
Chairperson, Peer Assistance for Chemically Dependent Nurses Committee
SR2, Box 6B
Madison, VA 22727 (home);
or
UVA Hospitals
Box 405
Charlottesville, VA 22908
(804) 924-5888 (daytime)
(703) 948-6694 (evening)

Washington State Nurses Association

Washington State Nurses Association maintains a list of nurses willing to assist their chemically dependent peers. A position paper on the "Need for Employee Assistance Programs for Chemically Dependent Nurses" has been written. A continuing education class dealing with the subject of chemically dependent nurses is presented periodically. An audiotape, "Reaching Out: Nurses Share Recovery," a discussion with a group of recovering nurses, is available for $10.00, with discounts available on quantities.

Contact: Cherie Clausen, M.N., R.N.
Coordinator, Educational Services
Washington State Nurses Association
83 South King Street, Suite 500
Seattle, WA 98104
(206) 622-3613 (daytime)
Hotline: (206) 622-3613. Available 8:00 a.m.-5:00 p.m., Monday-Friday.

West Virginia Nurses Association, Inc.

Nurse Care Network is a voluntary peer information and support network for nurses suffering from problems such as: addiction, stress, burnout, and others, with a strong emphasis on post-treatment individual and group support. Education and prevention information, seminars and workshops are provided to nurses, supervisors and students. The Nurse Care Network is endorsed by, but not sponsored by, West Virginia Nurses Association.

Contact: Barbara C. Banonis, B.S.N., R.N., O.P.C.
Chairperson, Nurse Care Network
Barbara C. Banonis Associates
P.O. Box 8491
South Charleston, WV 25303
(304) 342-5110 (daytime/evening)

Wisconsin Nurses Association

The Wisconsin Nurses Association Board of Directors on July 21, 1988 took action to establish a task force to further explore a peer assistance program for nurses whose practice is impaired by substance abuse. The task force will include representatives of WNA, the WNA Economic and General Welfare Commission, and ten other nursing organizations in the state.

Contact: Nancy Cervanansky, M.S.N., R.N.
Chairperson,
Peer Assistance Task Force
Wisconsin Nurses Association
6117 Monona Drive
Madison, WI 53716
(608) 221-0383 (daytime)

Wyoming Nurses Association

Wyoming Nurses Association is currently investigating options related to peer assistance. Because of limited resources, WNA is currently able only to refer nurses whose practice is impaired by substance abuse to treatment programs in the state.

Contact: Mary Lou Scavnicky-Mylant, Ph.D., R.N.
Box 306S
University Station
Laramie, WY 82071
(307) 766-4291

Appendix II: Agencies and Professional Groups Concerned with Substance Abuse

SPECIALTY NURSING GROUPS

American Nurses' Association
Committee on Impaired Nursing Practice
2420 Pershing Road
Kansas City, MO 64108

Drug and Alcohol Nursing Association
13 W. Franklin Street
Baltimore, MD 21201

International Nurses Anonymous
c/o Patricia Green, M.S.W., R.N.
1020 Sunset Drive
Lawrence, KS 66044

National Consortium of Chemical Dependency Nurses
99 West 10th, Suite 319
Eugene, OR 97401

National Nurses Society on Addictions
2506 Gross Point Road
Evanston, IL 60201

IMPAIRED NURSE NETWORK

The NNSA Impaired Nurse Committee maintains a network of contacts across the country that are available to assist nurses to get in touch with resources. It facilitates nurses in contacting other nurses interested in the issue of nursing impairment as well as to help recovering nurses contact each other. The network may be utilized by contacting the Chairperson, Pat Green, or one of the committee members listed below. All nurses with an interest in impaired nurses are encouraged to become a part of the network by sending information to one of the committee.

IMPAIRED NURSE COMMITTEE

Pat Green, Chairperson
1020 Sunset Drive
Lawrence, Kansas 66044
(913) 842-3893 (home)

Deanna Alexander
2105 Westkendal Lane
Arlington, Texas
(817) 461-0655 (home)
(817) 930-7822 (work)

Lee Byroads
4885 Kane Street
San Diego, California 92110
(619) 275-2610 (home)

Betty Harakal
2865 NE 13th Ave.
Pompano Beach, Florida 33064
(305) 942-7436 (home)
(305) 785-3938 (work)

Trisha Pearce
P.O. Box 22582
Seattle, Washington 98122
(206) 324-2419 (home)
(206) 583-4344 (work)

Nancy Guptill
40 Ellsworth Road
Peabody, Massachusetts
(617) 531-0496 (home)
(603) 899-2808 (work)

Nancy Miller-Cross
2448 Golden Gate Avenue
San Francicso, California
94118-4316
(415) 386-3014 (home)

Anne Catanzarite
4263 Losco Rd. #1425
Jacksonville, Florida 32223
(904) 359-6331

OTHER AGENCIES AND PROFESSIONAL GROUPS

Alcohol and Drug Problems
Association of North
America
Suite 181
444 North Capitol Street, N.W.
Washington, D.C. 20001

American Bar Association
750 North Lake Shore Drive
Chicago, IL 60611

American Council on
Alcoholism
Medical Center Suite 16-B
300 East Joppa Road
Baltimore, MD 21204

American Dental Association
211 East Chicago Avenue
Chicago, IL 60611

American Medical Association
535 North Dearborn Street
Chicago, IL 60610

American Medical Society on
Alcoholism
12 West 21st Street
New York, NY 10010

American Pharmaceutical
Association
1015 15th Street, N.W.
Washington, D.C. 20005

Association of Labor-
Management Administrators
and Consultants on
Alcoholism
1800 North Kent Street, Suite
907
Arlington, VA 22209

Association for Medical Educa-
tion and Research in
Substance Abuse
Career Teacher's Center
Box 129
Downstate Medical Center
Brooklyn, NY 11203

Center for Alcohol Studies
Chapel Hill, NC 27514

Center for Professional Well
Being
5102 Chapel Hill Boulevard
Durham, NC 27707

Center of Alcohol Studies
Rutgers University
Smithers Hall
Piscataway, NJ 08854

Drug Enforcement Administration
1405 Eye Street, N.W.
Washington, D.C. 20537

International Commission for the Prevention of Alcoholism and Drug Dependency
6830 Laurel Street, N.W.
Washington, D.C. 20012

National Association of Alcoholism Treatment Programs
2082 Michelson Drive, Suite 304
Irvine, CA 92715

National Association of Social Workers
7981 Eastern Avenue
Silver Spring, MD 20910

National Association of State Alcohol and Drug Abuse Directors
Suite 530
444 North Capitol Street, N.W.
Washington, D.C. 20001

National Association on Drug Abuse Problems
355 Lexington Avenue
New York, NY 10017

National Clearinghouse for Alcohol Information
16C-10 Parklawn Building
5600 Fishers Lane
Rockville, MD 20857

National Clearinghouse for Drug Abuse Information
10A-43 Parklawn Building
5600 Fishers Lane
Rockville, MD 20857

National Council on Alcoholism
12 West 21st Street
New York, NY 10010

National Institute on Alcohol Abuse and Alcoholism
16-105 Parklawn Building
5600 Fishers Lane
Rockville, MD 20857

National Institute on Drug Abuse
10-05 Parklawn Building
5600 Fishers Lane
Rockville, MD 20857

Oregon Institute of Alcoholism Studies
Willamette University
900 State Street
Salem, OR 97301

Pharmacists Against Drug Abuse
Welsh and McKean Roads
Spring House, PA 19477

University of California at San Diego
Summer School of Alcohol and Other Drug Studies
UCSD Extension
X-001
LaJolla, CA 92093

University of Utah School on Alcoholism and Other Drug Dependencies
P.O. Box 2604
Salt Lake City, UT 84110

Index